VAXBABY
The Curious Parent's Guide to **Pediatric Vaccines**

by Forrest Maready

Feels Like Fire
Wilmington, North Carolina

Text copyright ©2019 by Forrest Maready
Cover are & typography ©2019 by Forrest Maready

All rights reserved, ©2019. Published in the United States by Feels Like Fire, an imprint of Feels Like Fire.

No part of this book may be transmitted or reproduced in any form by any means with permission in writing from the publisher. Besides historical references, the names, places, and accounts mentioned in this book are used anonymously. Any resemblance to actual persons, living or dead, is entirely coincidental.

Printed in the United States of America

Library of Congress Cataloging-in-Publication Data
Names: Maready, John Forrest, author.
Title: Vaxbaby.
Subtitle: The curious parent's guide to pediatric vaccines.
Description: Wilmington, North Carolina : Feels Like Fire, [2019]
  | Includes bibliographical references and index.
Identifiers: Library of Congress Control Number: 2019911130 (paperback) | ISBN 978-1092641548 (paperback)
Subjects: LCSH: Vaccination in children. | BISAC: MEDICAL / Immunology.

Feels Like Fire
www.feelslikefire.com

Also by Forrest Maready:

The Autism Vaccine, 2019
Unvaccinated, 2018
The Moth in the Iron Lung: A Biography of Polio, 2018
Crooked: Man-made Disease Explained, 2018
My Incredible Opinion Vol. 2, 2017
Massa Damnata, 2017
My Incredible Opinion Vol. 1, 2016

Table of Contents

The U.S. Pediatric Vaccine Schedule ... 7
The First Thing You Should Know About Vaccines ... 11
Pregnancy: The TDaP & Flu Shots ... 16
How to Decline Vaccines if You're Pregnant ... 23
Should You Get a Rhogam Shot? ... 27
Should Family Members Get Vaccines? ... 30
The Hepatitis B Vaccine ... 34
What About the Vitamin K Shot? ... 39
Your First Well-Child Visit ... 43
The Pertussis/Whooping Cough Vaccine ... 46
The Tetanus Vaccine ... 52
The Diphtheria Vaccine ... 55
The One Chart That Changed Everything ... 58
Do Vaccines Actually Work? ... 63
Should You Be Concerned About Vaccine Ingredients? ... 67
The Polio Vaccine ... 73
The Hib Vaccine ... 79
The Pneumococcal Vaccine ... 83
The Rotavirus Vaccine ... 86
The Vaccine Schedule ... 89
The 4-Month Checkup ... 92
The Flu/Influenza Vaccine ... 95
The 9-Month Checkup ... 99
The Measles Vaccine ... 101
The Mumps Vaccine ... 105
The Rubella Vaccine ... 107
The Chickenpox/Varicella Vaccine ... 109
The Hepatitis A Vaccine ... 112

VAXBABY: The Curious Parent's Guide to Pediatric Vaccines

The Disease You Should Fear Most	114
How Natural Immunity Can Be Better	118
Are Vaccines Safe?	122
Why Vaccine Makers Can't Be Sued	127
Will Your Doctor Fire You?	130
How to Find a Flexible Doctor	134
Should You Sign Vaccine Refusal Forms?	138
Vaccines If Your Child is Sick?	140
Should You Spread Shots Out?	143
Can Your Children Still Attend Public School?	147
The Meningococcal Vaccine	151
The HPV Vaccine	155
What If Your Doctor Tells You Differently	159
What About Herd Immunity?	164
Should You Give Your Children Tylenol Before/After Shots?	170
What About Autism & Vaccines	173
Are Vaccines and Allergies Related?	179
What Kind of Side Effects Do Vaccines Cause?	182
Can Your Children Be Taken From You?	186
How To Recognize Vaccine Injuries	189
Don't 3rd World Countries Need Vaccines?	192
Should You Be Worried About Zika?	195
Closing	200

The U.S. Pediatric Vaccine Schedule

Pregnancy
The Flu/Influenza vaccine
The Pertussis/Whooping Cough vaccine
The Diphtheria vaccine
The Tetanus vaccine

Birth
The Hepatitis B Vaccine
The Vitamin K shot

2-month Checkup
The Hepatitis B Vaccine
The Pertussis/Whooping Cough vaccine
The Diphtheria vaccine
The Tetanus vaccine
The Polio vaccine
The Hib vaccine
The Pneumococcal vaccine
The Rotavirus vaccine

4-month Checkup
The Hepatitis B Vaccine
The Pertussis/Whooping Cough vaccine
The Diphtheria vaccine
The Tetanus vaccine
The Polio vaccine
The Hib vaccine
The Pneumococcal vaccine
The Rotavirus vaccine

6-month Checkup
The Hepatitis B Vaccine
The Pertussis/Whooping Cough vaccine
The Diphtheria vaccine
The Tetanus vaccine
The Polio vaccine
The Hib vaccine

The Pneumococcal vaccine
The Rotavirus vaccine
The Flu/Influenza vaccine

9-month Checkup

The Hepatitis B Vaccine
The Polio vaccine
The Flu/Influenza vaccine

12-month Checkup

The Hepatitis B Vaccine
The Hib vaccine
The Pneumococcal vaccine
The Polio vaccine
The Flu/Influenza vaccine
The Measles vaccine
The Mumps vaccine
The Rubella vaccine
The Chickenpox/Varicella vaccine
The Hepatitis A vaccine

15-month Checkup

The Hepatitis B Vaccine
The Pertussis/Whooping Cough vaccine
The Diphtheria vaccine
The Tetanus vaccine
The Polio vaccine
The Hib vaccine
The Pneumococcal vaccine
The Flu/Influenza vaccine
The Measles vaccine
The Mumps vaccine
The Rubella vaccine
The Chickenpox/Varicella vaccine
The Hepatitis A vaccine

18-month Checkup

The Hepatitis B Vaccine
The Pertussis/Whooping Cough vaccine
The Diphtheria vaccine

The Tetanus vaccine
The Polio vaccine
The Flu/Influenza vaccine
The Hepatitis A vaccine

4-6 Year Checkup

The Pertussis/Whooping Cough vaccine
The Diphtheria vaccine
The Tetanus vaccine
The Polio vaccine
The Flu/Influenza vaccine
The Measles vaccine
The Mumps vaccine
The Rubella vaccine
The Chickenpox/Varicella vaccine

11-12 Year Checkup

The Meningococcal Vaccine
The Pertussis/Whooping Cough vaccine
The Diphtheria vaccine
The Tetanus vaccine
The Flu/Influenza vaccine
The HPV Vaccine: Gardasil/Cervarix

16 Year Checkup

The Meningococcal Vaccine
The Flu/Influenza vaccine
The HPV Vaccine: Gardasil/Cervarix

Chapter 1
The First Thing You Should Know About Vaccines

Congratulations on making this investment in you and your family. I expect this book may play a big part in shaping the decisions you make about child's health. By now you've realized there's a lot of information out there regarding all the different facets of raising a healthy child: what to feed them, how they should sleep, how to discipline them. These days, there are growing numbers of parents who are putting more effort into researching vaccines. When I was a baby, they weren't such a big deal—I might have gotten four or five of them. Nowadays, health officials in the United States are suggesting children receive over 70 vaccines by their teenage years—many of them for diseases you've probably never heard of.

I can understand why this makes a lot of new parents nervous. If you are a mother, you are asked to make all sorts of changes to your lifestyle during pregnancy to ensure your baby has the best environment in which to form. You probably started eating organic, stopped drinking alcohol and all sorts of other modifications. After you've given birth to a perfectly healthy baby, it might feel odd to start injecting them right away with a bunch of pharmaceutical products.

While some people are opposed to all vaccines, no matter the situation, others have skipped or delayed particular vaccines for certain children. You may have already delayed a well-child visit because your child was sick. Everyone is different. Some people feel like there are too many shots (I'm definitely one of those people), while others may choose to follow a more lenient vaccine schedule from another country such as the Netherlands. Still others may skip booster shots for a previous vaccine because their child reacted poorly to the first one. Some folks don't have a problem with the 72 vaccines children are suggested to receive in the United States and would have no problem if many more were added. The next few chapters should help you make clear, confident decisions about where you fit in.

If you're like most people, right now you're trying to figure me out. You want to know where I stand, right? Am I pro-vaccine, or am I anti-vaccine? You want to know where I stand so that you can interpret what I'm saying with the right filter. I'd want to know the exact same thing, so I'm going to tell you precisely where I stand. For now, here is the best way to think of me: I want fewer vaccines—as few as possible. I'm constantly trying to figure out how to provide a healthy upbringing for my family with the fewest vaccines possible. Zero would be ideal. That's the truth about me in a nutshell—every bit of research and questioning I do is in an attempt to minimize the vaccines my family needs.

I'll talk more about ingredients later, but just understand that I think of vaccines like chemotherapy. You'd probably never give your child chemotherapy *before* they had cancer, even if you were told it might protect them if they happened to get it later on in their life. Why? The chance of them getting cancer is so low, you'd probably rather not expose them to the trauma of chemo in the off-chance they might need protection in the future.

You may think this is a poor analogy because chemo is much worse than vaccines. I thought that too, at first. The side-effects of chemotherapy stop soon after you stop taking them, but vaccines are different. Because they're designed to alter your immune system forever, the side effects of something going wrong can last for a very long time. As a result, I take the risk/benefit analysis of vaccines very seriously.

Here are the main factors that might go into my decision to delay or skip a certain vaccine: What's the chance of my child contracting the infection? What's the chance of permanent harm from the infection? What's the likelihood the vaccine will actually be working *when* they're likely to get that infection? And finally, what's the chance of permanent harm from the vaccine?

There are very few people who randomly decide to forego vaccinations for themselves or children. Unless they were raised in a family that didn't vaccinate, most people spend hours researching the risk versus the benefit of certain vaccines and infections before they make a decision to skip a single one.

After considering these factors, there are growing numbers of people who are deciding to delay, skip or avoid certain vaccines altogether. Some of them are refusing all vaccines—even the big ones like polio. As it turns out, polio was one of the first shots I decided to knock off my personal vaccine schedule. If you're shaking your head in confusion or anger right now, that's okay! Hang on to that thought for just a few minutes—the stories we've been told growing up make it seem dangerous to skip some of these vaccines. Once you start looking a little deeper into the actual facts, you'll realize the story is a bit different than you were likely told.

Before we really get started, I want to share a quick story with you. In 1916, New York City declared the first week of May "Baby Week." The sanitation and nutrition of babies in the city were horrible, and many died before their first birthday of illnesses like tuberculosis or diarrhea. So doctors, nurses, and health officials decided to make an effort to educate parents on the importance of cleanliness for good health—things you and I would probably consider basic rules of sanitation: Don't leave dirty diapers lying around your house for weeks at a time. Don't dump trash out of your window onto the street. Don't bathe your baby in the same water you use to clean your cookware. It may seem crazy these sorts of things had to be taught, but cramming thousands of people into apartments—people who had previously been living in rural countrysides—created a bunch of problems most people had never had to deal with. In the country, fresh water was often plentiful. Reusing water for different things in the city was as much because of necessity as it was ignorance.

Health officials had a contest to name "the best baby in all Greater New York" and on Sunday—what they called "Baby Sunday"—a prayer was read in churches throughout the city. This prayer is especially significant because although they didn't realize it at the time, much of the medical care children received at the time was as deadly as were the sanitation problems. Pregnant women, ill with morning sickness, would often be prescribed arsenic. Yes, arsenic. Children sick with anything, including teething, would be prescribed mercury—in the form of powder. They'd keep increasing the dosage of mercury if it didn't make them feel better until they started foaming at the mouth—that was the sign doctors were taught to look for to let them know they were at the maximum dosage.

As you take a closer look at vaccines, it's helpful to understand the horrible conditions children from the 1800's and 1900's grew up in. It wasn't only overcrowded conditions and horrible sanitation. The medical care was just as bad. So before we begin, I want to take you back to that Sunday in May, 1916, New York. I want to read that prayer to you that was read aloud to all of the new parents and soon-to-be parents across the city. Hear these words, and take them to heart as you make your way through this book:

> O, God, since Thou hast laid the little children into our arms in utter helplessness, with no protection save our love, we pray that the sweet appeal of their baby hands may not be in vain. Let no innocent life in our city be quenched again in useless pain through our ignorance and sin. May we who are mothers or fathers seek eagerly to join wisdom to our love, lest love itself be deadly when unguided by knowledge. Bless the doctors and nurses, and all the friends of men, who are giving of their skill and devotion to the care of our children...
>
> Forgive us, our Father, for the heartlessness of the past. Grant us great tenderness for all babes who suffer, and a growing sense of the divine mystery that is brooding in the soul of every child. Amen.

Chapter 2
Pregnancy: The TDaP & Flu Shots

If you've just become pregnant, an incredibly complex sequence of events has begun to take place within your body. You, no doubt, have sensed the changes but behind the scenes, adjustments to your hormones and immune system are happening to ensure your baby develops properly and is safe from harm. You might not feel very good, but you can rest assured these changes are temporary and are meant to protect the precious life developing inside of you.

One of the most interesting changes takes place within your immune system. You are growing a new life inside of you after all and without some changes, your body would consider it an invader. To prevent your body from rejecting anything, your immune system is being suppressed in a specific way so that your baby is welcomed and given everything it needs.

Another fascinating change most people aren't aware of: Initially, the brain overdevelops. You may recall how our brains are made up of a complex matrix of neural connections. As your baby's brain develops, this matrix is actually too dense. During the last few weeks of your pregnancy and the first few weeks of your baby's life, hormonal and immunological changes help prune their brain to the correct state.

If both of these processes sound intricate or complex to you, they are. In fact, they seem even more intricate and complex to those who study them—so elaborate that most scientists will freely admit they don't understand how they work. How your body develops a foreign life system, doesn't reject it, but instead feeds it and keeps it safe from sickness is still a mystery to those who research it. The way an infant's brain over-develops initially but then gets pruned back at just the right time is another component of fetal growth that we're still trying to understand.

There are many other parts of how you are able to perfectly form a baby that we don't understand—these are just two of them. We know a lot, that's for sure. We know a lot more than we used to, but we have no idea how much we *don't* know. Because of this, doctors tend to be very careful about the sorts of things women who are pregnant are told to do. Certain activities might be restricted. Certain foods or drinks might be banned. And if you've ever been prescribed medicines, you will probably remember many of them having those little stickers on them that say "Do Not Take If You Are Pregnant."

Why do medicines have this label? For the most part, because they've never been tested on pregnant women. And why is this? Because it's considered too dangerous—not worth the risk. And because they haven't been tested on pregnant women, the manufacturers that make certain medicines, the doctors that prescribe them, and the pharmacies that sell them all work together to make sure these products aren't taken by women who are pregnant. Even if the mother is very sick, her doctor might recommend she avoid taking a particular medicine for fear of what it might do to her developing child.

When you're pregnant, your doctor will most likely recommend you get two injections to protect your developing baby. These are the flu shot and the TDaP shot—what many just call a tetanus shot. The TDaP shot actually contains three vaccines: tetanus, the T in TDaP, diphtheria, the D in TDaP, and pertussis, the P at the end. Because they'll also recommend a few doses of a slightly different form of this shot for your child starting at their 2-month old checkup, I'll cover the details of this injection in a later chapter.

The reason the TDaP shot is recommended is really for only one of the three vaccines—the P, or pertussis, also called whooping cough. They don't really care about the other two—tetanus or diphtheria—it's just the pertussis they're concerned with. The hope is that because of the shot, your immune system will generate antibodies and pass them along to your infant so that when they're born they'll already have some protection from whooping cough before they get their own shots—something which could happen in utero or through breast-milk once they're born.

Should you take this shot while you're pregnant? If it were me, I would never allow them to inject me with this shot. Again, I talk more about pertussis/whooping cough in a later chapter, but for now I would skip this shot. Why? For starters, they don't really know if a shot given to a pregnant woman can cross the placenta and give protection to the baby. Why don't they know this? Because similar to other medicines, the TDaP shot has never been tested on pregnant women. Why? Because it's considered too dangerous. Vaccines are different than normal medicine. They're powerful products designed to create immunological changes in your body that last a very long time. If they don't work perfectly—which sometimes happens—the effects they might cause may last for years. If a medicine doesn't work or causes a problem, you can stop taking it and the negative effects will go away quickly. Vaccines don't usually work this way. They're meant to last a very long time so their side effects can also last a very long time.

This shot wasn't recommended to pregnant women until recently. Just a few short years ago, doctors wouldn't have dreamed of injecting pregnant women with nearly any medicines—never mind a vaccine. What happened? Was there an outbreak of whooping cough in 2-month old babies that scared people so much they decided to make a change, despite the risks? No. There was no outbreak. There wasn't an increase in deaths. There was no dramatic event that happened that caused doctors to start doing this. There were certainly no safety studies performed that convinced them it would be safe. The recommendation was made from a medical organization, without any safety data, and doctors started doing it.

If you've never looked into vaccines, you will probably have a hard time accepting that your Ob-Gyn would recommend anything that might be dangerous for your baby. Normally, they wouldn't. For some reason, this recommendation of the TDaP vaccine has been accepted as okay despite it having never been done before and despite it never having been safety tested. Your doctor may tell you they've injected hundreds of women with the vaccine and haven't seen any problems. That may be true, but the reality is it would be impossible to tell the reason a woman miscarried or their infant developed problems months later. When doctors say they've never seen any problems, what they really mean is they've never *personally associated* any problems they've seen with the vaccines they've administered to pregnant women.

You're probably asking, well what's the risk from the disease? What's the risk of going that two months after birth before my infant can get the shot themselves? I'll talk about that in the pertussis chapter, but for now, just know that this shot started being recommended not because babies were being harmed by the infection, and not because it was decided to be safe based on some extensive studies being done, but simply because they thought it would probably be safe. As I mentioned before, the shot has two other vaccines included you and your baby will also need to deal with—whether you want to or not. In the past, you may have heard of someone getting a single tetanus shot but it is near impossible to get a standalone version (or the pertussis vaccine) in most countries.

There is a lot more to talk about for this shot and infection but as I said before, if I were pregnant, I would never in a million years allow anyone to inject this shot into me and my fetus. We don't understand a hundred things about developing babies during pregnancy, and we certainly don't understand how this shot might affect them. Mothers have safely delivered millions of babies each year for time eternal without this shot.

What about the flu or *influenza* shot? Like pertussis, the flu shot has recently begun to be recommended for pregnant women. Doctors would've never dreamt of injecting such a product into pregnant women a few decades ago but without any safety testing being done, they started recommending it in 1997. You can look at 25 different flu shots that are licensed in the United States and you'll see that not a single one of them has been safety tested in pregnant women.

You might think that if they're safe for humans then they should be safe for infants. This may seem logical, but there is something important you should know: Pharmaceutical companies like to think of babies as "little humans." In fact, they are very different. They're not adults with a smaller dosage requirement.

Infants have incomplete kidneys. They have incompletely developed brains. The immunological relationship between the mother and her fetus is very unique and unlike anything scientists can create in their labs. It is foolish to assume safety tests on adult humans can be transferred onto developing infants and babies, albeit on a smaller scale. They're *very* different than fully-developed adults in many ways other than their size.

This difference has been made obvious in a few studies that have associated various forms of the flu shot with a heightened risk of miscarriage. Of course those who make and recommend the flu shot to pregnant women will downplay the risk, but knowing the fragile balance the mother's immune system must maintain with what would otherwise be considered a foreign invader, it's not surprising that a product purposefully designed to manipulate the immune system might occasionally confuse things.

The flu shot is widely known to be a mediocre shot. It has never worked well and manufacturers are always struggling to guess the right strain for the upcoming season. The reality is that the influenza virus is constantly mutating—it doesn't just mutate once during the offseason then maintain that form for the next 12 months. It's constantly changing and to develop a shot that works against it well is near impossible. You may have heard people joke about getting the shot, then getting the flu, but that's not because the manufacturers guessed the wrong strain—it's because of something completely different. The shot depresses a particular component of the immune system that protects you from getting sick and can make you more susceptible to other infections, like RSV, otherwise known as respiratory syncintial virus.

Until recently, most flu shots contained mercury—a poison so toxic you're instructed to avoid eating fish by your doctor while pregnant. Strange they considered it safe to inject for years when they were so particular about you *not* ingesting it in your food. While most flu shots don't have mercury in them anymore, a few still do. Regardless of whether it has mercury or not, I would avoid it like the plague if I were pregnant.

As you will soon see, it's not always the ingredients that matter so much. A lot of new moms will try to make an ingredient list of each vaccine to determine if they're comfortable injecting those ingredients into their infants based on the risk from a potential infection. The reality is many vaccines activate your immune system in ways that differ from a natural infection and can cause future problems that don't really have anything to do with the ingredients themselves. If it were me, I'd skip any vaccine during pregnancy, unless there was some strange life-threatening situation I can't envision right now.

Chapter 3
How to Decline Vaccines if You're Pregnant

If you're pregnant and the thought of TDaP or flu shot doesn't sit well with you—or if the fact they've never been safety tested in pregnant women and weren't even recommended until recently makes you uncomfortable—you can decline these shots. I want to give you a few pointers about how to do this so nobody's feelings get hurt and everyone is happy.

It's a shame this chapter is even necessary. In a perfect world, your Ob-Gyn and their nurses would respect your decisions and not give you any trouble. Unfortunately, some may offer resistance. As you know, vaccines are a contentious topic and many doctors and nurse's feelings get hurt when you question their advice. Some even become aggressive or downright mean when questioning your decision.

For you to suggest you're not interested in the flu shot or TDaP shot while pregnant suggests to them they're wrong for all of the other women they've administered the shots too. Some mothers will do their research, print out studies that indicate these shots aren't safe for pregnant women, and will hand them over to support their decisions. Depending on your relationship with your doctor, I wouldn't always recommend you do this. These scientific papers can come across as arrows—weapons that basically say "you're wrong to administer these shots to pregnant women and I have proof."

The number of mothers refusing these shots is growing by the day, and many doctors or nurses dread yet another pregnant mother—who may have no formal medical training—implying their standard practices are harmful. The reality is you've likely spent more time studying the cost/benefit of a maternity vaccine than they have and your research is likely to highlight this.

The best time to handle this situation is while you're interviewing various Ob-Gyns, ideally before you are even pregnant, or have just become pregnant. Let them know right away you're likely to decline any unnecessary medical procedures during your pregnancy for the safety of your baby. Ask them if they have a problem with that. Ask them if they have any problem if you decide to decline the flu or TDaP shots.

Emphasize that you've made a personal decision, based on either research you've done or the advice of other people in your life that you trust. Certain physicians or nurses may be tempted to debate you. Unless you're an aggressive personality and enjoy this sort of thing, I'd avoid getting drawn into arguments. They're unlikely to change their mind about anything in that setting and will likely take your stance personally. Your choices are a personal decision that they have absolutely no business trying to manipulate. Let them know you're not interested in debating the pros and cons and are happy to send them studies later if they're interested in understanding why you reached the decision you did.

If you're able to have this conversation earlier in your pregnancy rather than later, it will typically go better. If you sense the employees at a particular practice are not going to respect your wishes, it is a safe guess they will give you pushback on other decisions you want to make later in your pregnancy. These two vaccines are important decisions, but they're not the only ones you will need to have support on from your physicians and nurses.

A quick note about something most people don't realize: Vaccines take a little bit of prep work to get ready. They may require mixing and for those stored in refrigerators, they may need time to reach room temperature. Once they've been prepared, they need to be administered within a certain timeframe or else they'll need to be thrown away. When you go into an appointment where the doctor or nurse is likely to offer you these two shots, they'll have already begun this prep work ahead of time so everything will be ready. When they've already prepared the vaccines and you decline, this may create another bit of tension. Save them—and yourself—the trouble by letting them know ahead of time that you won't be needing any vaccines. When you first meet with your Ob-Gyn, ask them at which visit they will recommend the flu and/or TDaP shots so that you can call them ahead of time and remind them not to draw up any vaccines for you.

Finally, take someone with you. I'll mention this again elsewhere, but there is absolutely nothing wrong with taking your spouse or trusted friend along with you to help support your decision. Many new mothers aren't prepared for someone who aggressively challenges their decision with threats of horrible things happening to their baby if the mother won't do as she's told. This is a very sad development in recent years as more mothers have begun to question vaccines. Medical professionals can sometimes respond very unprofessionally. They're in their comfort zone in the doctor's office and often have no problem issuing veiled threats of harm if you don't listen to them. Because of this, I'd take someone with you to these types of appointments to help support you in your decision. It can feel extremely lonely with a physician and one or two nurses staring you down with laser eyes as you try to defy their demands. I hate that some doctor's appointments have turned into this kind of tension, but unfortunately the medical community does not take kindly to their most popular procedure being questioned.

If you have a spouse or mother who is not *completely* on board with your decision, I wouldn't recommend taking them with you. They will also feel the peer pressure of doctors and nurses and will likely suggest you listen to their demands in order to diffuse the tension.

To summarize, I would make up your mind *before* you go to this appointment and stand by it. Don't attempt to debate someone or argue with them. It will likely not go well. Just hold firm that you have made a personal decision and don't feel the need to convince anyone else they're wrong with theirs. They will typically move along if they don't feel personally threatened by your decision.

Chapter 4
Should You Get a Rhogam Shot?

If you're pregnant and are being recommended the Rhogam shot, you may have questions about whether this procedure is necessary or safe. The Rhogam shot is often given to mothers with a negative blood type at 28 weeks and within 72 hours of birth. You probably remember how there are different blood types: A, B, AB and O. Sometimes you'll hear blood types mentioned as *A positive*, or *A negative*. That negative or positive indicates your Rh factor. If a particular protein is present on your red blood cells, you're Rh positive. If your blood type was B, they'd say you're B positive—your blood is in the B group *and* you're Rh positive. B negative would mean your blood is in the B group but you're missing that special protein on your red blood cell. You're Rh negative. About 82% of people are Rh positive. The rest are Rh negative. Being Rh negative doesn't make you unhealthy but can cause a problem under a very rare circumstance.

If you're pregnant and have a negative Rh factor, doctors are going to recommend you receive a shot, possibly two, of Rhogam. Let me explain why. If the Rh factor of your fetus is Positive, and for some strange reason their blood mixes with yours, you can develop antibodies to that Rh positive blood. Your baby's blood will be seen as an invader by your immune system because theirs has that special protein and yours doesn't. What would cause this mixing of blood? Well it would be a very rare event: Trauma from a car wreck or other accident. Rarely, a miscarriage or amniocentesis might trigger it. Regardless of what caused it, that initial event—what's called a *sensitization event*—is harmless. Your blood now recognizes Rh positive blood as an invader and has antibodies to it. The end. The problem happens if one of these blood mixing events happens *again*, a second time. This doesn't have to be with the same baby, but a future pregnancy. If you have another baby and they also have Rh positive blood, and *another* one of these blood mixing events happens, then there can be a problem. The antibodies in your blood can attack theirs, because it sees it as foreign. Obviously, the likelihood of this happening is almost nothing, but if it does happen, it can be really bad. It can cause stillbirth, or babies to be born with what is called Rh disease.

The Rhogam shot is really similar to a vaccine. It contains the same Rh positive antibodies (from other humans who we assume were screened properly) you would produce if Rh positive blood happened to mix with yours. The hope is it will trick your body into thinking it doesn't need to react to the invading Rh positive blood because your body will believe it has *already* reacted to them.

This should seem a bit odd. If one of these traumatic events hasn't happened to you, why would you purposefully create the result of the event? Essentially, what they're saying is "A mixing event might cause you to create Rh positive antibodies, so to avoid that danger, we'll just inject them on purpose ahead of time." So what happens if you just received a Rhogam injection and there is a traumatic event? Well, because of the injection, you now *already* have Rh positive antibodies in your bloodstream which can mix with your baby's blood and cause problems. The injection just skipped you past Step 1, which posed no danger, and took you straight to Step 2, where there can be a problem.

In Europe, this shot is administered directly after pregnancy, when blood is likely to mix. This works fine. They have no epidemics of Rh diseased babies dying in the womb or shortly after birth. After the baby is born, the shot poses no danger to them. If I was Rh negative and miscarried, I would probably consider getting the shot immediately. If I was Rh negative with a positive baby, and needed to perform amniocentesis, I might consider getting the shot. Otherwise, I would skip it during pregnancy. It has as much chance of harming your Rh positive baby as helping in the event your blood mixes. And if it hasn't already been mentioned to you, if you and the father are *both* Rh negative, your baby should be Rh negative and you will have nothing to worry about, no matter the situation.

Chapter 5
Should Family Members Get Vaccines?

You may have heard that family members who are going to be in contact with your baby should get vaccinated. There are thousands of different viruses and bacteria that can be spread from person to person. Most of them have no vaccine available. While a few of them do have a vaccine available, many of them do not prevent the spread of the disease.

This is a strange concept to understand, and even many of the government health websites don't appear to get it. The main vaccine doctors will recommend family members get is the TDaP shot—the same tetanus, diphtheria and pertussis, or whooping cough, shot they recommend you get while you are pregnant. The reason they want your family members to also get it is because of something they call "cocooning." If everyone around your baby is protected from a particular disease, they argue this will then protect them in a cocoon of immunity.

While this sounds like a beautiful concept, it doesn't work that way, particularly with the TDaP shot. First off, tetanus is not a contagious disease. Despite the fact this bacteria exists all over the planet, it is *not* spread from person to person. Diphtheria, the D in the TDaP shot, is contagious but a very rare disease in countries with modern sanitation and hygiene. The pertussis component of the shot, for whooping cough, is the main reason doctors will tell you to have your family members vaccinated before they can see your child.

The problem with having your family members vaccinated for this infection is very serious. The vaccine for pertussis, the P in the TDaP shot, does *not* prevent the spread of the infection. Let me say that again: The whooping cough shot does *not* prevent whooping cough from spreading. It simply minimizes the uncomfortable symptom, which is coughing. The bacteria which causes whooping cough is not affected by the vaccine. The shot is designed to protect you from the poison the bacteria can make, not the bacteria itself.

If you get a pertussis infection, it may be mild, but it will make you cough. If you get a bad infection, you will cough *a lot*. This is a warning sign from nature. Its purpose is to let you know to stay away from young children. If you're a parent of a small child and someone is coughing violently near your child, you would naturally take them away. If you yourself were coughing violently, you'd probably not feel good about picking up a little infant. Why? You'd know you might get them sick.

If you get the TDaP shot and the pertussis component works (not always a given), you may not experience this vigorous coughing as a warning sign for yourself and others to pick up on. You may have a pertussis infection, but you will have *no* idea. This is not good. The result is you may pick up that infant who is actually vulnerable to a pertussis infection without realizing you are about to infect them. Imagine having a collection of black widow spiders and using a black Sharpie to paint over the red hourglass figure on their backs. If someone were to see this spider, they'd have no idea it was capable of injecting them with a poison and causing them serious harm.

In the same way, the TDaP shot covers up nature's warning signs of whooping cough so that infections spread undetected. Because of this, if my family had a new infant, I would insist that family members *not* get this shot. I want them to *know* they're sick. I want them to experience that coughing—a clear indication that they should stay away from my baby.

There are a few other shots—those that contain live viruses—that can actually spread after you get vaccinated. The main source of paralysis from the poliovirus in many countries is now the vaccine itself. Why? Because the virus in the vaccine occasionally gets loose and causes problems. When everyone is getting the poliovirus vaccine, chances for accidents are higher.

This is the reason if you go to a cancer ward, you'll sometimes see a sign that forbids people from entering who've been recently vaccinated. Some cancer patients undergoing chemotherapy have suppressed immune systems and shouldn't expose themselves unnecessarily to any risk. To do that, administrators may ask people who were recently vaccinated to avoid contact with these patients. This is a rare event, but the risk is enough that hospitals will try to keep the recently vaccinated away from their most sick patients.

The science on which vaccines can "shed," which is what the phenomenon is referred to, is not clear. Some articles will say vaccines don't shed at all, but admit you might get an actual infection from the vaccine, which will cause you to accidentally infect someone else. This is basically a word game which attempts to confuse people into believing vaccine shedding doesn't exist. The reality is, vaccines do shed. This is why they just removed a particular strain of poliovirus vaccine in India—because it was causing more paralysis than the naturally occurring virus was. The vaccines known to shed are MMR (measles, mumps, rubella), chickenpox or the Varicella shot, the shingles shot (which is not a pediatric shot), and the influenza or flu shot. If I had an infant, I would ask anyone that was going to come in contact with them if they'd recently had any of those shots—and by recent I would mean in the last two or three weeks.

It's probably strange to hear this—a completely different take on having relatives around you vaccinated to help protect your child. If you doubt what I'm telling you, that's good—start doing some more research on the subject and once you find actual scientific studies on the issue, you'll realize that these are simple phenomenon that are easily explained and that public health officials and physicians aren't super happy about admitting.

So if someone tells you to tell your mother or mother-in-law to get the TDaP shot for whooping cough to protect your baby, I'd tell them no thanks and that you'd prefer to be able to tell if someone is sick or not.

Chapter 6
The Hepatitis B Vaccine

Okay, the big day is here. Your beautiful baby is born and placed on your chest for a chance for you to bond. Before long, they're taken away for a "bath" and testing. While you might believe these procedures are necessary for birthing a child in the hospital, the first vaccine they'll likely recommend your baby receive is something you really ought to take a close look at.

Hepatitis B is a viral infection that can be passed from an infected mother to her offspring. The infection can occasionally persist in certain people causing liver problems like cancer—often decades later. Hepatitis B is not very contagious and is most commonly spread through IV drug use, blood transfusions, or what is termed risky sexual contact, like prostitution. Most women who are pregnant are tested for hepatitis B. No matter if you test negative or positive, the hepatitis B vaccine will be strongly suggested for your infant.

Some countries, such as Denmark, Sweden and Iceland don't allow *any* vaccines in the first three months of a child's life. It's thought the protective antibodies of the mother's breastmilk shouldn't be interfered with and offer the best immunization a baby could have. Many other countries don't recommend the hepatitis B vaccine for infants unless the mother has tested positive. In the

United States, they'll recommend your infant receive, within hours of birth, the hepatitis B vaccine, no matter what. Why is this? Is it necessary? Is it safe?

The hepatitis B vaccine was originally designed for people at high risk of developing liver problems—IV drug users, people with risky sexual lifestyles, and those who'd received multiple blood transfusions. As you can imagine, this is not a very big pool of people to market to, and vaccine development is very expensive. Because mothers positive with hepatitis B can pass the infection onto their children, it was thought these children could benefit from such a vaccine. It didn't take long before public health officials in charge of vaccine schedules decided to include all infants for the hepatitis B vaccine, just in case the testing mothers received during their pregnancies missed something. This may strike you as odd, and it should. I'm going to go ahead and tell you the truth about something right here. As a new mother, you really need to hear this part: In the United States, where many vaccines are manufactured, the pharmaceutical lobby is extremely powerful. It's the most powerful political group in the world. They exert a tremendous amount of pressure on health officials to add vaccines to the childhood schedule. They do this for a couple of reasons. One, it provides free sales they don't have to advertise for. Two, other countries often follow the United States' lead. And three, manufacturers can't be sued for problems with their childhood vaccines—they're protected by the government.

Hepatitis B liver cancer deaths were not killing massive amounts of children (or adults for that matter). Pediatric hepatitis B infections were not soaring out of control—the virus isn't really contagious in the normal ways. The vaccine was created for a small population and through some aggressive political lobbying was added to the childhood vaccine schedule. It's really that simple. The vaccine was not created because parents were begging for a medical intervention to a horrible child killer. Most parents have no idea what the disease even is. Yet in the United States, this vaccine is administered to hours old infants every day. To add to the problem, the vaccine has never truly been tested to see if it works. Although they test for the presence of antibodies to the virus after vaccination, they can't test to see if the vaccine actually prevents someone from getting an infection. That would be considered unethical. So we can't do a real test to see if it works, just a half-measure that doesn't truly tell us if the vaccine even works. Kind of crazy, but unfortunately, true.

If the vaccine was a simple product with no risk, perhaps it wouldn't be that bad. But in addition to being grown in animal organs, it contains a large amount of aluminum. I'm going to go into depth explaining the problem with aluminum in a few other chapters, but for now, just know that aluminum is a neurotoxin and is possibly the last thing I would want to inject into my children. Vaccine manufacturers don't *want* to put aluminum in their shots but they don't work very good without it. So they add the aluminum and we're stuck with the effects. Without going too far down the rabbit hole, just know that aluminum is being implicated in Alzheimer's disease, autism, and some autoimmune disorders. These are all diseases that appeared around the same time we started adding aluminum to vaccines. Whether they're the cause or not, we don't know yet—scientists have never really looked. They've studied mercury quite a bit, but never aluminum. So while we wait for research to explain why the brains of adults with Alzheimer's, the children with autism, and the intestines of those with Crohn's disease, seem to have so much aluminum, I personally will steer as far away from aluminum as I possibly can. I'll repeat this a couple of times throughout this series, but there is no disease on the planet I fear more than the effects of injected aluminum.

In my personal quest to reduce the number of vaccines my family needs, the hepatitis B vaccine is the easiest one to skip, especially if I was the mother and had tested negative for a Hepatitis B infection. If you decide to skip this vaccine, you will want to tell the nurses ahead of time, and in fact, you will want to watch your baby like a hawk. Nurses administer this vaccine so frequently, they're likely to forget you asked them not to do it. If it were me and I had to give birth in a hospital, I wouldn't let them take my infant away from my sight unless my child's life was in danger. They will jab your child with this ridiculous vaccine so fast they won't even remember having done it. I've talked to several mothers who swore their child never got an infant hepatitis B vaccine but were shocked to look through an itemized chart of their maternity bill from the hospital and find it listed amongst other things.

Here's a quick hint if you want to skip this shot for your newborn: Try and not make a big deal about it. You should let them know early on, maybe as part of your birth plan, that you don't want this vaccine for your infant. Don't try and make them feel wrong for administering the vaccine to other infants, or bring in scientific research papers. Just tell them you want to wait until you see your pediatrician for any vaccines to be administered. Finally, you should be very careful in the hospital. Unfortunately, I've heard of nurses administering the shot outside the room and not telling the mother about it. They will want to remove your baby for a bath and have plenty of opportunity to sneak it in then. This is why many women end up working with a birthing center, midwife, or doula—

they can be pleasant birthing experiences where your wishes—and not the hospital's—are the most important.

Chapter 7
What About the Vitamin K Shot?

Directly after you give birth, you'll be presented with two potential injections for your infant. The first is the hepatitis B vaccine and the second is an injection of Vitamin K. This isn't a vaccine at all but an injection of a synthetic vitamin to help prevent your baby from developing internal hemorrhages. This is a very rare occurrence and I'll explain more about that in a minute, but just know that vitamin K helps create proteins that allow blood to clot properly. Babies are born with low levels of vitamin K and as a result can bleed more aggressively than a normal person might—kind of like people who are on blood thinners.

If a baby develops a problem, it's usually internal where doctors are unlikely to notice it right away. Because of this, since 1961, doctors have been injecting newborns with a synthetic form of vitamin K in hopes the extra boost would promote more aggressive blood clotting and prevent any injuries—however rare they might be—from happening.

Should you allow your infant to have this shot? While the vitamin K shot does contain a tiny amount of aluminum, and I mean tiny—like way, way less than any vaccine, that's not what concerns people about it. It contains a large amount of benzyl alcohol, something that has been shown to affect liver function.

Some people think this is why so many babies seem to be born with jaundice these days—yellow skin that often indicates a temporary liver problem. If you get a vitamin K shot, that benzyl alcohol may interfere with your baby's liver, causing them to develop jaundice.

The main reason I'd be reluctant to administer this shot to my infant is because of the humility I've developed over years of medical research. There is so much about the human body that we don't understand. Because of a decades old piece of research that noticed babies had lower amounts of vitamin K than normal humans, doctors immediately assumed this was a problem that needed to be corrected. You've heard the saying everything is a nail when you have a hammer? It seems like as humans if we notice a pattern—like infants have lower vitamin K than adults—we automatically assume this is an error that we should correct. The reality is we *don't know* enough to say whether this deficiency might be part of nature's grand design. For decades anyone with intestinal surgery would have their appendix removed just because we didn't understand how it worked. It appeared to our limited context to not be necessary. Now we are beginning to fully understand why the appendix is in fact a very important organ to our gut health and those who had it so callously removed are suffering the consequences.

In the same way, we don't really know if infant vitamin K levels are low *on purpose*. Like their kidneys, an infant's liver doesn't work as effectively as an adult's. The result is it can't convert or store vitamin K as well. There may be a very specific reason for this we are unaware of. Just a decade or two ago, you would've been laughed at for suggesting the appendix might have a use we were unaware of. They aren't laughing now. Knowing that U.S. infant mortality rates are among the highest in the industrialized world makes me begin to feel like maybe mother nature had things figured out just fine for the last million years.

The vitamin K shot does appear to work. There is no doubt about that. Vitamin K promotes blood clotting, and if you have more of the vitamin, your blood will clot more easily. No real mystery there. But here's something that will really get your blood boiling. There is an infant oral vitamin K—one without the benzyl alchohol—but it's not available in many countries. If it's in a syringe and can only be administered by a doctor, they'll move heaven and earth to get it approved and mandated for every child born on this planet. If it's in a medicine dropper and can be bought over the counter, then pharmaceutical lobbyists will exert extreme pressure, saying things like, "Maybe we shouldn't let parents decide if this is right. They might get the dosing wrong. They might forget to complete the treatment."

If you're set on supplementing your child's diet with vitamin K, there are organic drops available from retailers. They won't mention any infant usage, because they don't want to get sued, but I know many mothers buy them for their infants. For reasons I won't go into now, I'd avoid the drops that have any form of Vitamin D added to them—go for just the vitamin K alone. You'll have to do a little research online to find a dosing regimen you feel comfortable with.

Apart from the questionable ingredients and incomplete understanding of the human body, I have problems with any injections unless they're absolutely necessary—something I'll explain in a later chapter. If it were me, I would *not* give my infant the vitamin K shot. I realize that it works, but I would be very concerned about injecting benzyl alcohol and its effect on their underdeveloped liver. If I was really nervous about it, I'd get some oral vitamin K drops and do that instead.

Chapter 8
Your First Well-Child Visit

Before you attend your first well-child visit, I want to give you a heads up on something you may not know. This is a bit of a summary of some other topics I cover more in detail. If you don't have a support network of more experienced mothers around you, you may have a lot of questions about your infant at this appointment. Your doctor will probably be able to answer all of them—*unless* those questions are about vaccines. Because the number of mothers who are questioning vaccines has exploded, doctors can be less than thrilled to have another mother in their practice who might question the wisdom of their most tried and true procedure. It'd be like getting pulled over by the police for speeding and asking them, "Are you sure you even know how to write a ticket?"

For most pediatric doctors, vaccines are the most important medical procedure they have. Other mothers have come in before you, and will have asked the same questions you might ask: Do these shots contain aluminum? Have you ever had any problems injecting all of these vaccines at the same time? I hate to have to say this, but these sorts of questions are likely to make them mad. Not only are you questioning their most common procedure, but by skipping or delaying certain vaccines, you can cost them a serious amount of money. I explain this in a later chapter, but just know that if the doctor catches a whiff you may be questioning the vaccine schedule at all, their blood pressure may shoot through the roof. They may even try to threaten you by asking you to sign an official looking "vaccine refusal" form—I also talk about what to do about that in a later chapter.

The last thing I want to mention real quick is about the prep work that goes into getting vaccines ready for your visit. Before your appointment, a nurse has to complete a couple of steps. Vaccines are usually stored in refrigerators, sometimes in different parts. Sometimes they have to be mixed together before hand and allowed to reach room temperature. Once this happens, they must be used within a short period of time or they will have to be thrown away. At a busy doctor's office, this isn't such a problem, but you can imagine why an overworked nurse, who busted her butt to get seven or eight vaccines ready to go for your appointment while she was doing all of her other tasks, you can see why she might get a little miffed to walk into your appointment and realize that she had wasted her time for nothing and now has eight vaccines that need to be used on someone else so they don't have to go in the trash.

Between this and having one of their foundational procedures being questioned by someone who didn't spend tens of thousands of dollars on their medical education, it is unsurprising these well-child visits don't go as well if you have some hesitancy about vaccines.

What do you do with all of this? Simple. If you have questions about vaccines you want to ask your doctor, don't do them at a visit when vaccines are expected to be administered. Do it before hand. Schedule an appointment with the specific purpose of getting your questions answered. If you go walk into an appointment with questions about vaccines and there are eight vaccines sitting in a tray on the table beside him, you are not likely to have a productive conversation. If your doctor won't let you schedule an appointment for this purpose, let them know ahead of time that you don't want any vaccines at the 1st well child visit. Tell them not to prepare any vaccines, because you have a few questions, and aren't sure you are ready to move forward with the procedure. If you get there and they're already drawn up, they will try to exert tremendous pressure on you so the vaccines don't get wasted. You really don't want to deal with that pressure when you have some serious questions you need answered.

Bring someone with you who agrees with you *completely*. Many new mothers get bullied into vaccinating their children by aggressive doctors or nurses. They'd done all their research, and felt like they were ready to take on the world, but caved to the pressure in the doctor's office. Because of this, I'd recommend you take someone with you to this appointment who will help support you in your decision.

Remember, unless you are completely comfortable at your first well-child visit with your baby receiving up to eight vaccines, call them ahead of time and let them know not to prepare the vaccines. They may reveal a little bit more about their character than you intended on seeing, but regardless, your visit will go much better this way.

Chapter 9
The Pertussis/Whooping Cough Vaccine

At your 2-month well-child visit, your doctor will measure your baby's length, weight and head circumference. They'll ask about any concerns you might have, and will expect to administer another dose of the hepatitis B vaccine. If you didn't read the chapter on the hepatitis B vaccine already, I'd go back and read it now. Hepatitis B is a vaccine originally intended for adults at high risk of this obscure illness and was never intended for babies. Outside of the U.S., most other countries do not recommend this shot for infants. The next shot they'll recommend your baby receive contains a vaccine for pertussis, or whooping cough.

Pertussis is the P in the DTaP shot, the shot which contains vaccines for diphtheria, tetanus, and pertussis. You may have noticed I said TDaP for the vaccine they recommend while you're pregnant, and DTaP for your baby. This is not a typo. There are two slightly different mixtures of this vaccine. The TDaP shot—the one that starts with a "T"—is the one they normally recommend for anyone who is teenager or older. The DTaP version of the shot is for everyone younger than a teenager.

Whooping cough is the result of a bacterial infection. The bacteria produces a toxin that causes inflammation and liquid to build up in the lungs. It's called whooping cough because of the sound children make when they have this infection. I've seen plenty of videos of children with whooping cough and they've never sounded like "whoops" to me, but instead more like the bark of a little squirrel. Anyway, out of all the infections we vaccinate for, this is actually the only one that I worry about. All of the other ones are so rare you are never likely to encounter them—vaccinated or not. Pertussis is a bit more common. Not as common as the flu or a cold, but pertussis infections do happen and when they do, they can cause babies trouble. Let me explain why.

Adults and children really don't have a problem with whooping cough. As I said, inflammation from the toxin the bacteria produce cause your lungs to become irritated. This creates a lot of mucus. You have to get this mucus out of your lungs and the way humans do this is by coughing. Coughing forces the liquid out so that you can breathe more easily. Babies, especially infants, can't cough very well. They don't have the muscle tone built up in their abdomen or diaphragm to really cough hard so they're not able to get that liquid out as easily. If they don't get the liquid out, it can cause them breathing problems and they can develop pneumonia, which is never fun.

Once they're a few months old, your baby can cough and they're likely past the danger point. It's never fun to see your baby coughing wildly with an infection—it can be really scary. No one wants their baby to have a whooping cough infection. But we do know about ways to minimize your baby's discomfort if they were to get an infection. You can give them large doses of vitamin C, something which will make the mucus very watery. This makes coughing it out much easier for a young infant. After you've done this, you can actually hold them at an angle and the liquid will sometimes just run out of their lungs. Again, there is really a small window of time after their born before they can cough it out themselves that you need to worry about, but it is something to learn how to recognize and deal with right away.

You can look on the internet and find some videos that moms have posted of their children with whooping cough. They've done this to help other moms who are thinking of skipping the pertussis vaccine see how to recognize whooping cough and also to see how the coughing isn't always as bad as some people might imply. If you see a news article about whooping cough, they will often find a baby who has pertussis but hasn't been treated with anything to make the mucus more watery. They will definitely struggle to get the mucus out, and it looks awful. If you know how to recognize it and know how to help your infant with vitamin C and possibly some rotated postures, it can be fairly trivial. Look for some videos online and you'll see what I'm talking about.

You're probably wondering, if pertussis can be kind of scary, then why on earth wouldn't anyone just give their child the vaccine? Like I said, pertussis is really the only infection I'd worry about if I had an infant less than three or four months old. Why not just give them vaccine and not have to worry? I wish it were that easy—I really do. We all want things to have simple answers. Doctors will tell you, give your child the DTaP vaccine and everything will be fine. No worries.

The reality of the pertussis vaccine is not very pretty. I talk more in depth about this in another chapter, but you should know that the pertussis shot doesn't try to protect you from pertussis bacteria itself, but a toxin the bacteria produces. What this means is you can still spread the bacteria to other people, even if you just had the vaccine three weeks ago. So having your family members vaccinated for whooping cough to protect your baby doesn't work. In fact, it's actually really dangerous because if they get the vaccine and become infected, they won't cough so bad. That coughing is nature's signal for you to keep your baby away from them, and if they're not coughing—because of the vaccine—you'll never know they're in danger. Because of this, I would actually plead with my family members not to get any vaccines before my baby arrived.

Another problem with this vaccine is that it doesn't work that well. Obviously, even if your child has the vaccine they can still get the pertussis infection, but sometimes the protective effect against the toxin doesn't even work and they still have that coughing problem. This can be dangerous because many parents just trust that their infants are completely fine—they had their vaccines, after all when, in fact, their baby might actually be in danger. As you become a vaccine-aware parent, you'll realize that you are the greatest protector of your child's health, no matter their vaccine status. You'll learn the symptoms you can safely ignore and the warning signs you might need to take action with. People tend to think if you go to all your well-child visits and get your 72 vaccines you never have to worry about your child having any health problems. Unfortunately, the reality is much different.

Here's another problem with the pertussis shot. If you've heard of how overuse of antibiotics can cause new strains of a bacteria to emerge, it's become apparent the pertussis vaccine is doing the same thing. A new strain of the pertussis vaccine has recently emerged, one that the vaccine does not work for. It's like playing whack-a-mole with these different microbes. If you push down here, another one pops up over here in its place. Nothing is free. Everything has a cost. Vaccines have a cost. Antibiotics have a cost. And I'm not talking about money, I'm talking about deferred illness. You pay now, or you pay later, and as my father used to tell me, it's *always* more expensive later.

Because this is such an important decision, I want to mention an obscure part of vaccines and immunity that may interest you. If you have a daughter, and she gets a pertussis infection naturally, she will generate true lifelong immunity. She will never have to worry about getting the infection again, and she won't be able to silently spread the disease like a pertussis vaccine-recipient might. Additionally, when she has children, she will be able to pass this immunity onto them through placental transfer and breast milk. Those initial two years of her children's lives will be protected through the illness she caught while young. Vaccines don't work this way. You cannot pass on vaccine protect the way natural immunity does. This is a strange concept to think about, because I would never purposefully infect my child with pertussis, like people used to do with chickenpox or mumps. However, if your daughter were to get infected, she would be able to grant an immunological gift to her children. Nature has a way of turning struggle into steel —it makes you stronger, even your children stronger. Amazing.

Finally, the pertussis vaccine is part of a shot called DTaP. It used to be called DPT. It had a P instead of the "aP." The "a" stands for acellular. The original DPT vaccine really seemed to have an association with SIDS and some other neurological problems, so they decided to try and make a safer version of it. The reason we think it could have been so dangerous is because the pertussis bacteria has a unique ability to breach the blood brain barrier—a protective lining that keeps bad things from getting into your brain. Nowadays, researchers purposefully use the pertussis bacteria to get past this protective barrier. The new vaccine was supposed to have reduced this effect. Unfortunately, the DTaP vaccine—the one your child is suggested to receive 5 times—is still associated with some of these problems. Like the tetanus and diphtheria components, it contains aluminum, an ingredient I would never inject into my family unless there was a deadly outbreak of disease that appeared uncontainable, even with aggressive quarantine. I will explain the particulars of aluminum in a later chapter, but just know that out of all the questionable ingredients in vaccines, this is the one that terrifies me the most. It's not the polysorbate 80, it's not the formaldehyde, and it's not even the occasional mercury preservative thimerosal. It's aluminum and the pertussis vaccine—along with the other two components of the DTaP shot—all contain aluminum. There is no disease on this planet I fear more than the effects of aluminum. Medicine can treat most any type of infection there is. Medicine has almost no answers for the devastation aluminum can cause.

Because there is such a tiny window of time where I wouldn't be thrilled about my infant getting a pertussis infection, and because there are ways to deal with it if it did happen, and because the vaccine contains a large amount of aluminum, I would never consider giving anyone in my family this vaccine. The chances it would work are too low to justify the potential negative effects of its ingredients.

Chapter 10
The Tetanus Vaccine

Another vaccine that will be recommended for your child at their 2-month well-child visit is the tetanus shot—the T in DTaP. Tetanus is an extremely rare illness, with or without a vaccine. Tetanus bacteria tends to be found outdoors, usually in areas where cattle or horse manure have been. The bacteria are harmless anywhere in your body except your nervous system. If you were to rub it all over your skin, even your mouth, nothing bad would likely happen. It's only when tetanus bacteria get in your nervous system that they can cause problems.

People associate tetanus with stepping on a rusty nail, but it doesn't have anything to do with rust or metal. It lives in the fecal material of certain animals. If you get cut by something that has some cow dung on it, then there is a less than 5% chance you may get a tetanus infection. If you do, there is something like a 90% chance you fight it off naturally with no drama. It's once in a blue moon that it actually causes neurological problems. Besides, there are ways to treat a wound so that there is essentially zero risk of a tetanus infection.

Tetanus never came close to killing people like some of these other diseases, even during the height of the metallic medical malpractice days. Total numbers of tetanus infections—not deaths, but infections—were only in the hundreds at the worst. DEATHS from tetanus were never very high. It was extremely rare to die from this infection.

This vaccine was added to the childhood vaccination schedule not because children were dying from tetanus, but because they could. In the 1930s, children were receiving the diphtheria vaccine and manufacturers, who also made the tetanus vaccine, thought "Hey, let's just combine these together and children will never have to worry about diphtheria or tetanus ever again."

At the time, parents *were* concerned about diphtheria, but not tetanus. It was so obscure, even most children running around barefoot on farms weren't ever told by their parents about the dangers of stepping on rusty nails or anything like that. The vaccine was added because it was easy, it could make a few extra bucks, and it was thought it might save a few kids from a tetanus infection.

Unfortunately, the tetanus vaccine contains aluminum. I mention this in the some of the other DTaP chapters, but the tetanus, diphtheria, and pertussis shots don't work very well without aluminum. When they added aluminum to the shots in the 1930s, their marketing materials insisted that only one shot would be necessary with the aluminum-containing shot. As it turns out, the tetanus vaccine, like the diphtheria and pertussis vaccines, don't work well—even with the aluminum—so now your kids are supposed to get it five times and there is talk of adding a sixth.

If my odds of getting a diphtheria infection were 1 in a 100 million, and tetanus is even lower, *and* the vaccine contains aluminum, *and* I'm supposed to give it to my child 5 times, then no way—there is no way I would give this shot to my child, for the *hope* it might work years later if they were to get a 1 in a 100 million infection. If your kid were playing on a farm and stepped on a rusty nail and you were convinced they were going to get a tetanus infection, you can always get a Tetanus immune globulin shot—if that event were to happen. An immune globulin shot isn't a vaccine but something more like anti-venom you might get after a snake bite. Until then, there is no way I would ever let my child have a tetanus shot.

Chapter 11
The Diphtheria Vaccine

Diphtheria is another vaccine your infant will likely be recommended at 2-months old. It's the "D" component in the TDaP vaccine. Diphtheria is a bacterial infection that causes a white, leathery coating on your tongue and throat and like a lot of bacterial infections, it's not the bacteria itself that's the problem but a type of poison we call a *toxin* the bacteria produces which causes the symptoms. Interestingly, most people get a diphtheria infection and never even know it—it's just some that seem to react to it negatively and generate massive amounts of these toxins.

With a diphtheria infection, the white leathery coating on the tongue or throat can get so thick it will make breathing and eating difficult—especially for young children—and in really bad infections, the toxin can sometimes travel through your blood and cause respiratory or breathing problems. Diphtheria could be contagious and was typically spread by coughing or sneezing. It used to be a horrible disease and many children would die from it every year but it has all but disappeared from modern society. Some suggest your chance of getting a harmful diphtheria infection in a first world country is less than one in 100 million. This is not just because we have a diphtheria vaccine now, although it may have something to do with it.

A few scientists believe diphtheria has a kind of 100-year-cycle that ebbs and flows the way other infections might come and go with certain seasons. I believe a large part of the reason diphtheria infections were so deadly was the way they were treated by doctors —often with mercury or by burning off the patches in children's mouths with acid.

Regardless, diphtheria is now considered an infection easily controlled by proper sanitation and easily treatable by modern medicine, even if you happen to react to it horribly. If you have trouble breathing, doctors can intubate you—that is, they can put a tube in your mouth that keeps your airway open. They can also administer an antitoxin, the ingredient in the original version of the diphtheria shot. Antitoxins can counteract the effects of the toxin being produced by the diphtheria bacteria. They don't affect the bacteria itself, just the toxin they produce. Doctors can also administer antibiotics to get the infection under control. In first world countries, diphtheria is extremely rare, no matter the vaccination status of a group of people and it would be extremely odd for anyone to die from it because our physicians have gotten so good at treating it.

If the infection could be horrible in the past, but medicine can treat the infection fairly easily, you're probably wondering if you should get the vaccine for your child. Unfortunately, you can't make the decision as easily as you might like. The vaccine for diphtheria is only included with shots for tetanus and pertussis. Also unfortunately—they all contain aluminum, something I would never consider injecting into my child unless there was an epidemic of a deadly disease that appeared to be uncontrollable, even by aggressive quarantine.

Diphtheria was the first shot to ever get aluminum added to it —they did this because the original shot didn't work well and they had to administer three of them just to get any kind of protection. Back then, people didn't like giving their kids injections *at all* and weren't real happy about having to give their child three of them in hopes it would protect them from diphtheria. So aluminum was added and parents were promised this new vaccine was special because you only needed *one* shot. Not three, like the old one, but with the new vaccine—the shot that contained aluminum—you should only need one.

Well fast forward a few decades, and now your child will get five of them, whether you like it or not, because it's included with the tetanus and pertussis vaccines. And because the pertussis vaccine appears to be working so poorly, there is talk of adding a sixth. Parents may not be super happy about this, but vaccine manufacturers are probably thrilled.

Because this vaccine contains aluminum and the chances of getting the disease are one in a 100 million—and even if you did, medicine could easily take care of you—it's a no-brainer for me. If it were me, I would skip the diphtheria vaccine with zero anxiety or fear.

Chapter 12
The One Chart That Changed Everything

As I began to study vaccines, the single biggest surprise came in the form of a chart I saw in a book that had researched the history of vaccines. I'll never forget the confusion this chart created in my head. All my life I'd heard vaccines saved humanity from horrible things like smallpox and polio. Before vaccines, there was widespread death and destruction from disease. After the vaccines, all of the childhood illnesses that had plagued humanity for centuries disappeared—basically overnight. This is the chart that changed everything for me (from CDC data).

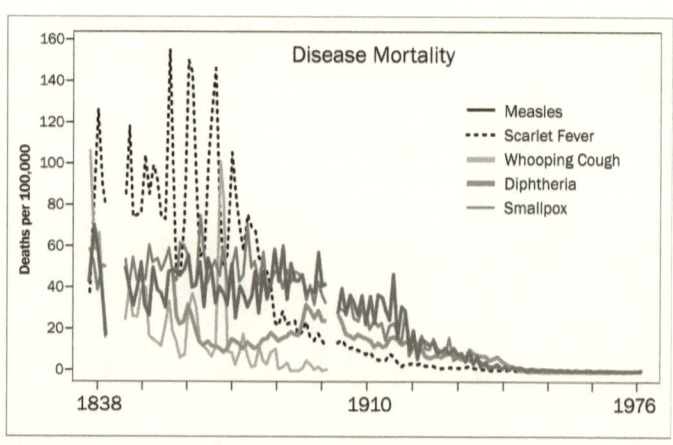

It showed how many people were dying from a couple of different diseases over the last 150 years. I couldn't believe what it suggested: every disease was getting less deadly *at the same time*. The thing that blew my mind was that one of the diseases didn't even have a vaccine. But it didn't matter—the mortality from all of them was going down in sync. I thought that either the data contained in this chart was fabricated, or the stories that I'd been told were wrong. The chart starts back at 1838, so there are some data gaps in places, but in general, the mortality from the 5 diseases on this chart were trending downwards well before vaccines were invented. I thought the author must have been using some statistical trick to look at deaths in a weird way that would get the result they wanted, but after a lot of investigation, I realized it charted deaths per 100,000 using government data sources.

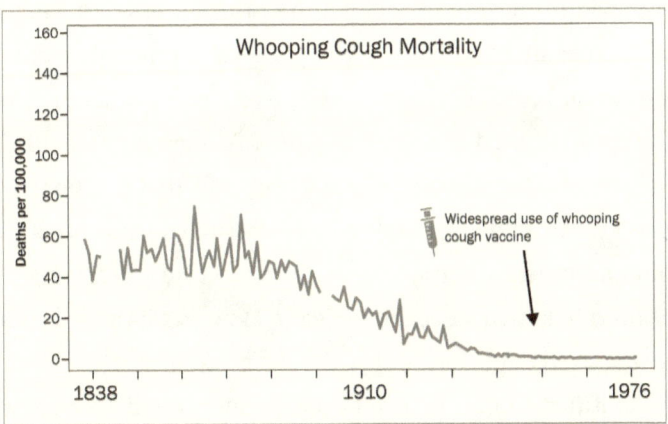

What was really shocking for me was pertussis, or whooping cough. The mortality from this disease was basically zero before the vaccine was even invented. Measles was the same way. These are two diseases that we still vaccinate for today and the mortality from them had fallen to nothing before the vaccine. Then the book pointed out the 5th disease on the graph—scarlet fever.

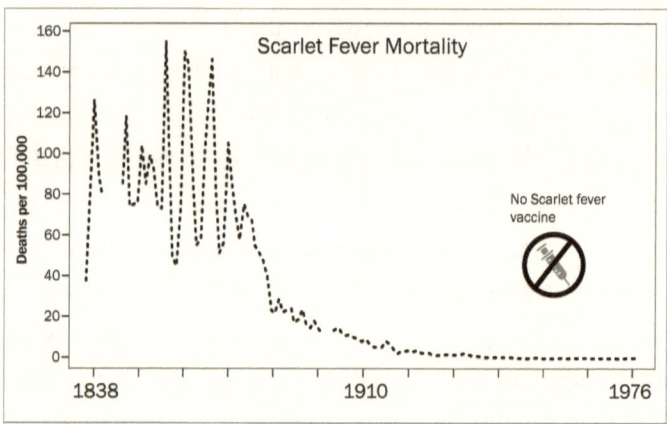

Scarlet fever is different than the others because they never developed a vaccine for it. Like the other diseases, it became less and less deadly over the past 150 years—even though it didn't have a vaccine at all. All of these diseases—plus many other ones without vaccines—followed a similar decline. I had grown up believing the smallpox vaccine eradicated smallpox, and that the polio vaccine saved kids from being paralyzed, so I assumed these other diseases would have a similar trajectory—horrible deaths before the vaccine was invented, then a decline in death. How was it these diseases had become so trivial before—or without—a vaccine?

As it turned out, people began to understand how disease was spread. If someone caught an infection, authorities could contain it by isolating that person and keeping them away from others. This meant disease outbreaks became far smaller. There were also improvements in food safety, hygiene, and sanitation that meant all of the health woes typical of life in the 1800s disappeared.

The biggest reason was the most shocking to me. All throughout the 1800s and into the 1900s, medical care was so horrible it often killed far more people than it saved. People began to realize that arsenic and mercury were probably not the best medical treatments to be giving infants and sick people. This move away from metals as a medicinal treatment helped save many sick people. Through improvements in living conditions and medical care, many of the diseases that were "killing" thousands of people eventually became trivial infections that no one feared—before most vaccines were even invented. You may have heard about a recent Johns Hopkins study that showed medical error to be the third leading cause of death in the United States. Heart disease and cancer are first and second, but medical error is in third place, killing 250,000 people a year. You may think that is horrible, and it is, but it used to be much worse. Many of the horror stories we've been told about various diseases were due to the absolutely horrible medical care people used to receive—even worse than today.

When I realized the mortality of all these different diseases began to come down at the same time, regardless of whether they had a vaccine or not, I felt like maybe I needed to rethink some things. I had heard stories of parents saying their kids developed autism soon after their vaccines, and I knew there were some rare side effects here and there. But if the diseases weren't really killing anyone, how bad were the vaccine's side effects? How often did they happen? Was SIDS really just a baby that died randomly with no explanation at all? Were food allergies really from ingredients in the vaccines like some people suggested? Everywhere I looked, the story was not the one I had been told as a kid, as an adult, or as a new parent.

Take a look at the chart and decide for yourself—either the chart is a lie, or maybe all of the improvements in medical care, sanitation and nutrition—maybe they had more of an impact on human health than anything else. If that is true, it ought to make you begin to question many other things you thought were true about vaccines.

Chapter 13
Do Vaccines Actually Work?

By now, you've heard a lot of information about vaccines. We grew up hearing vaccines saved us from certain death from all sorts of diseases. I've been showing you how the deadliness of most diseases plummeted around the same time *before* vaccines even became available. You're hearing two different things, and you're probably left wondering, do vaccines even work?

The answer is: Vaccines work—with an asterisk. Vaccines work—asterisk. They do their job. What is their job? To trick the immune system into developing antibodies for a virus, bacteria, or toxin, hopefully *without* causing nasty symptoms in the process. The asterisk is kind of a big deal, so let me explain what it's there for.

For the most part, I believe vaccines *can* do the little trick they were designed to do. They cause an immune response which can create the presence of antibodies. Antibodies are those things that attack the invader the next time your body recognizes it. It is a cheat—we all know that. Part of the reason it's a cheat is because we're injecting modified components of infectious disease directly into your body. Injections bypass many parts of your immune system that are meant to protect you—like your tonsils, your intestines, and your lungs. They create an immune response that's very different from just getting the infection naturally—one that doesn't really create true immunity. But, if you're looking for a very specific antibody, and take that as proof-positive the vaccine worked, well then yes, you could say the vaccine works.

Here's the problem. Because vaccines don't work the same way an infection does, the presence of disease antibodies doesn't equal immunity. It's different for each person. Scientists don't know why, but for many people, their response to a vaccine doesn't protect them from an infection. That's why you see stories where over 50% of people in a measles outbreak were vaccinated or 97% of people in a mumps outbreak were vaccinated. The vaccine may have "worked" for them in terms of generating antibodies, but it didn't work for them in terms of preventing them from getting infected.

Despite as many as 4 or 5 booster shots, they didn't develop immunity to the disease. They may have developed antibodies, but no protection. Some people don't even develop antibodies. The vaccine is completely pointless for them, other than perhaps a lifelong battle with eczema. They won't test whether a vaccine works by purposefully infecting someone with a virus or bacteria. So pharmaceutical companies must gauge a vaccine's effectiveness by looking at the number of antibodies created in response to it. For many people, and for reasons we don't understand, this measurement doesn't indicate whether they're immune or not.

Just so I'm clear, if the FDA tells drug companies their vaccine needs to be 95% effective. they'll say the vaccine is 95% effective if 95% of people in a test show antibodies for the disease. Now of course those tests can be manipulated to produce an acceptable number, but even so, amongst the group of people who *do* produce antibodies for the infection—whether it was an honest or fudged number—the percent of them who are actually protected from the infection is much, much lower. That's one of several dirty secrets that health authorities don't want to talk about. Look up the disease outbreak stories. You'll see how many are vaccinated- it's usually a majority of them. Disney measles—55% vaccinated. Texas High School measles—100% vaccinated. Harvard mumps—100%, vaccinated. If the MMR vaccine truly protected against 95%, then we should almost never see most of a measles outbreak occurring within people who were vaccinated for it. It's obvious when you start looking that many vaccines don't work anywhere near as well as advertised.

Finally, I want to point out a sneaky trick people who generate reports for these outbreaks sometimes do. If a report says 35% were "unvaccinated," that might mean 35% of people couldn't produce a record of their shots in time for the report to be published. It doesn't mean they never received any vaccines, it just means they couldn't find proof of their vaccination status. Sometimes, even if you can produce your immunization record but don't have all the recommended boosters, they'll still call you "unvaccinated." You might have an immunization card that says you got an MMR shot at 18 months and a booster at 4 years, but if your card doesn't show you got a third booster shot at 16 years old, you might be labeled unvaccinated.

Reports used to say x% were either unvaccinated or unsure of their vaccination status. Now, to hide how poorly vaccines work for some people, if you can't prove you've had every single booster shot required by the CDC, they will put you in the unvaccinated column. Just so you know, when you read these stories, there is a lot at stake behind the scenes with these numbers. Things frequently get manipulated so that vaccines look more effective than they actually are.

To summarize, vaccines can cause the immune system to create antibodies for an infection. But unfortunately, that doesn't come anywhere close to creating lifelong immunity for a disease. For a percentage of the population, vaccines can offer temporary protection from an infection. Protection in that case means you don't exhibit the traditional symptoms of the disease. You might still get infected, and you might still pass it on to your children, the elderly, and the immunosuppressed. Because vaccine protection and natural immunity are very different things, both in the way they protect, how long they last, and how they do or don't prevent the spread of the disease, I can say vaccines "work"s… but with a very large asterisk on the end.

Chapter 14
Should You Be Concerned About Vaccine Ingredients?

As people begin to research vaccines, most people start by focusing on the ingredients. If you didn't already read the previous chapter called "The One Chart," it shows how all the diseases began to decline around the same time—whether they had a vaccine for them or not. Make sure you read that first. It's scary to talk about ingredients because we've been so thoroughly trained to fear infections. If infections are universally bad, and vaccines contain ingredients we don't want to inject in our children, you're probably stressed out and thinking, "What should I do?" Just relax and keep listening. Knowledge is power, and in this case, knowledge will take away all of that stress and anxiety about disease and vaccines.

Like many pharmaceutical products, vaccines contain ingredients you wouldn't want to put in your children unless you had to. But it's a compromise, right? You take a small risk in the hope they're protected from a bigger risk. Unfortunately, vaccines do contain ingredients you would probably never consider feeding them if you were to look on their label. No one wants to inject their child with formaldehyde, polysorbate 80, or aborted fetal cell tissue. For now, I want to focus on an ingredient I mentioned in the hepatitis B shot—aluminum.

Many vaccines contain metals—on purpose, not by accident. Mercury has been a popular medicinal ingredient for two hundred years and was only recently recognized as being dangerous enough that it needed to be removed from vaccines. Mercury, or what's sometimes called thimerosal, is still occasionally used as a preservative in multi-dose vials of flu shots. Multi-dose vials are bigger and have a thin piece of rubber on the top called a diaphragm that keeps the vaccine inside free from contamination.

When a nurse or doctor draws up a vaccine by putting a syringe through the diaphragm in the vial multiple times, the chance of contaminating it with a foreign bacteria or virus increases. Thimerosal was added into these vaccines so if something got past the diaphragm, it would die because mercury is toxic to all forms of life—not a comforting thought for something you might inject into your child. Many vaccines used to come in multi-dose vials, because it was cheaper that way. Nowadays, most vaccines come in single-use containers and because they'll only be used once, you don't need the mercury anymore.

While Thimerosal has long been thought to cause neurological problems associated with vaccines, the danger of the *aluminum* they contain is only recently being understood. Aluminum is not a preservative—it serves a different purpose and is included in many vaccines regardless of whether they're in multi-dose vials or not. Aluminum has been in vaccines for a long time—since at least the 1930s—and its purpose is to aggravate your immune system into a stronger response. This is called an adjuvant.

When I say aluminum, you're probably thinking of aluminum cans being melted down into silver liquid and dripped into a vaccine. The aluminum used in vaccines is actually called a metal salt, and looks like a white, crystalline powder. It's still aluminum and is put in vaccines because your body hates it—your immune system reacts very strongly to it.

Because many of the components used in vaccines have been manipulated to the point they're less dangerous to inject, your body doesn't even see them as invaders and doesn't react to them. Aluminum is added because it forces your body to react to the vaccine. They don't want to put aluminum in there, but they have to. The vaccines will not work without it.

We've long known this aluminum to be dangerous. It's used in scientific experiments to help create asthma and food allergies in animals. It was shown as far back in 1921 to cause problems in your brainstem—a crucial component of your nervous system. The argument for their use has always been that vaccines contain such tiny amounts of aluminum that it couldn't be dangerous. People will tell you that you eat more aluminum every day than what is contained in vaccines. This is what people thought twenty years ago, but recent scientific research has made it clear why tiny amounts of aluminum in vaccines can be so harmful.

For starters, toxins that you eat, or ingest, rarely make it past your intestines. Although humans ingest a small amount of aluminum in their diet, only about .3% of it's actually absorbed into the body. Ingested aluminum is in an ionic form that's more easily filtered by adult kidneys and can be stopped from causing neurological damage. The aluminum that's injected with vaccines is in a different form called *nanoparticulates*. This form of aluminum is much different than the ingested kind and creates a couple of problems you will never see with the dietary kind.

If you were to take the aluminum contained in a single pediatric vaccine and inject it into a specific part of a child's brain, they would almost certainly die. The amount of aluminum in many of the shots children regularly receive is toxic enough to kill anyone if it was administered directly into the wrong spot.

Thankfully, this rarely happens. The safety with injected aluminum was always thought to be in its dilution. The dose might be deadly—we knew that—but it was assumed it was evenly distributed around the body rather than one specific place where it might cause serious problems. Think about pouring Kool-Aid powder into a pitcher of water. It spreads out on its own and only needs a little bit of stirring to mix it evenly throughout the water. We thought the ingredients of vaccines would spread out evenly throughout the body in that same way. Unfortunately, it turns out we were wrong.

Until recently, we made the logical assumption that the less aluminum the vaccine contained, the less of it might make it into dangerous areas of your body. We thought that if the amount of aluminum contained in the vaccine was so little, then the chance of a significant portion of the metal reaching your brain would be infinitesimally small.

An uncomfortable discovery about aluminum was made recently: less aluminum is worse. Less aluminum is *more* dangerous. In the study, researchers injected mice with varying amounts of aluminum. Across the study, mice who received less aluminum per injection fared worse—their behaviors indicated neurological problems and the amount of aluminum that reached their brain was much higher. The mice that received the two higher dosages of aluminum seemed to have less significant effects.

How could this be? When a vaccine is injected into your arm, the aluminum triggers an aggressive immune response and your body begins to mount an attack against it. This is often why your arm gets so sore after a vaccine—it's your body forming granulomas around the ingredients—a collection of fibrous tissue doing their best to wall off ingredients from the vaccine.

Scientists now understand that your body responds more aggressively with these granulomas at higher concentrations of aluminum. It makes sense when you think about it—the more dangerous the invader is perceived to be, the more aggressive the response. If you get a large dose of aluminum, the body works hard to wall it off inside protective granulomas. But the opposite scenario is more concerning—if the injection contains a smaller amount of aluminum, there is less granuloma formation and more of it makes it into your lymphatic system and blood. And if it gets into your lymphatic system and blood, it can get into your brain.

This was a stunning revelation that should've caused everyone to rethink what were safe amounts of aluminum in vaccines. Unfortunately, most health officials and physicians have acted completely unconcerned. Their websites have not been updated to reflect these new discoveries, and they'll shrug their shoulders if you mention it to them. If history has shown us anything, it's that those in authority will always be the very last to admit they were wrong. I wouldn't expect it to be any different with vaccines.

Manufacturers know aluminum is dangerous. They've been searching for an alternative for decades. Metals aren't the only questionable ingredients in vaccines that should make you think twice about injecting them into your children—there are a few others.

But for those of us committed to as few shots as possible, most of us would never allow aluminum-containing vaccines to be administered to our children. The chances of neurological injury from the accumulation of aluminum from these shots is simply too high to be worth the risk from any disease. With aluminum being so strongly implicated in the brain damage of autism and Alzheimer's, even certain autoimmune diseases, I wouldn't recommend anyone—children or adults—take any aluminum-containing vaccines either.

Chapter 15
The Polio Vaccine

At this checkup, your child will be offered an injected polio vaccine. There is another form of the vaccine which is given by mouth, sometimes on a sugar cube if you've ever seen the old pictures, but most likely your child will be offered the first of several *injected* polio vaccines. I became so fascinated with the polio story, I spent a few years researching it and wrote a book about it. After having researched polio more thoroughly than anyone I know of, I feel pretty confident I can explain polio and the vaccine to you.

Polio is probably the most famous disease we vaccinate for. Everyone can recall images of children in braces and people lying inside iron lungs before the vaccine. Anyone who grew up in the 1940s and 1950s probably knows someone in their family or neighborhood that was affected by this horrible disease.

As the story goes, in the 1950s a vaccine came along, and polio disappeared. You stopped seeing children in braces, and the iron lungs became a thing of the past. A heroic story of man over microbe that no one can deny, right? The truth about polio is not quite as simple as we were told and is actually more horrible than you can imagine.

Polio is a nickname for *poliomyelitis*, which means inflammation of the grey matter of the spinal cord. If you get a lesion on your spinal cord, that part of your body may develop paralysis. This disease nearly always occurred in children, which is why it was called infantile paralysis for decades. It almost always started in their legs, and as lesions continued to move up the spinal cord, they would lose control of their abdomen, their arms, and finally the muscles that expanded and contracted their lungs.

If they couldn't breathe, they'd die. The iron lung, first introduced in the late 1920s, helped children, whose lungs were paralyzed, to breathe. This was a godsend because some children could eventually recover from their paralysis—as long as they could keep breathing. The iron lung bought many of them enough time to survive until the lesions went away. They might have residual paralysis and difficulty walking but they would live. For some, they would go on to have completely productive lives.

Polio was basically non-existent before the 1800s. There might have been a case here and there, but you really don't see it in the medical literature until the 1890s when it began to appear in epidemic form. Some people will point to an Egyptian painting of a man with a cane and a shortened leg as evidence that polio always existed, but as you'll see, there is no way of knowing exactly caused this man's condition.

As it turns out, the paralysis of poliomyelitis can be caused by many different things. Several viruses can cause it, as can several different bacterial infections. Surprisingly, pesticides could also cause it. Studies were conducted in the late 1800s with a popular pesticide called Paris green. They purposefully fed animals too much pesticide and it paralyzed them in their "hind quarters"—just like what was happening with children. Scientists did autopsies on the animals, found lesions in their spinal cords, and pronounced they had died from poliomyelitis, or polio—from pesticide poisoning.

The pesticide contained a metal called arsenic, and may explain why many parents originally referred to polio as teething paralysis. A popular medical treatment at the time was "teething powders," a concoction given to infants who were teething. They contained massive amounts of a similar metal—mercury. Teething powders became popular in the early 1800s and appeared about the same time you start seeing isolated cases of polio. Coincidence? You decide.

It became clear that certain viruses and bacteria could also cause paralysis—but only if they got inside the nervous system. For all of human history, these microbes had never caused problems but starting in the late 1800s, they suddenly gained the ability to get into the nervous system.

This likely had something to do with a new pesticide that was invented in 1892—*lead arsenate*. It was a combination of lead and arsenic and was sprinkled and sprayed on many fruits and vegetables that were later eaten. It was extremely popular with farmers because it couldn't easily be washed off with water—which mean they didn't have to re-spray after a storm. For mothers trying to clean their children's food, this wasn't such a great invention.

It appears that not only did this metallic pesticide create paralysis directly through poisoning, but also caused a leaky gut issue in children that allowed different viruses and bacteria to pass through their intestines and into the spinal cord behind. Remember that humans had lived with these viruses and bacterial infections for hundreds of years with no paralysis until the late 1800s. Within a year or two of the invention of this new pesticide, polio began to appear in that same area of the country.

In the 1940s, at the end of World War Two, a new pesticide called DDT began being used by nearly everyone and polio became much worse. Unlike lead arsenate, which was sprayed on food, DDT was sprayed directly onto children in an attempt to protect them from flies and mosquitoes. Ironically, it was thought these insects could transmit polio, and DDT was sprayed on children to prevent the disease. Many people from this era will recall chasing the DDT truck down the street, playing in the clouds of pesticide trailing behind—another popular pastime that no doubt contributed to the paralysis of that era.

By 1952, people began to stop using DDT because many insects had already started to develop resistance to it. Parents also began to suspect it was more toxic than they'd been told. At the same time, cases of infantile paralysis, or polio, began to plummet. 1952 was the peak for polio cases in the United States—not just the kind caused by the poliovirus, but the paralysis due to all of the other viruses, bacteria, and direct pesticide poisoning. They all began to disappear as DDT stopped being sprayed on nearly everything.

Even though all types of infantile paralysis began to go away after 1952, most history books will say it's because of the Salk polio vaccine. This is just not true. The injected polio vaccine—the one we use today—worked horribly. It was officially introduced in 1955 but was quickly withdrawn because it was inadvertently causing paralysis due to manufacturing problems. Many didn't get a polio vaccine until years later, when a different, presumably safer version of the polio vaccine, the Sabin oral polio vaccine, came out in 1961.

By then, polio had all but disappeared from the United States. As it turns out, even the new vaccine wasn't actually needed. Polio had already nearly vanished. It had appeared suddenly in the 1890s alongside the introduction of the pesticide, lead arsenate, and had suddenly disappeared in the early 1950s alongside the abandonment of DDT. The story we grew up hearing left out many important parts. The paralysis of polio wasn't just caused by one virus, but many different things—all of them tied directly to the wreckless spraying of pesticides that began and ended in lockstep with the appearance and disappearance of polio.

I realize this may be very difficult for you to digest, but just to demonstrate the reality of what happened, I want to tell you about a scientific study that was conducted in Detroit in 1960. Because the initial polio vaccine worked so poorly, scientists were concerned. In an attempt to understand what was wrong, they took stool samples from almost 1,000 people who had been diagnosed with polio that summer. They tested all the samples and determined that less than one third of the people that were diagnosed with polio actually had an infection from the poliovirus. They had actually been paralyzed by one of the *other* viruses, bacteria, or possibly even acute pesticide poisoning.

This was the main reason the first polio vaccine wasn't working —the people didn't even have "polio" at all! They had been paralyzed by one of the many other causes of paralysis that appeared in the late 1890s and disappeared in the 1950s. It didn't matter that many of them had received 4 or more injections of the polio vaccine—they weren't paralyzed by polio, but something else, and the polio vaccine wasn't going to stop it.

Today, countries that still use dangerous pesticides like DDT continue to struggle with the paralysis we now call polio. They've controlled some of it with the polio vaccine, but remember, the vaccine only addresses a single cause of paralysis—the poliovirus. Because there are many other microbes capable of paralyzing, other forms of infantile paralysis have increased nearly just as much as poliovirus-caused paralysis has decreased. If they were to clean up their environment and stop using these dangerous pesticides, all forms of infantile paralysis would likely disappear just like they have in the United States.

This is why I would skip the polio vaccine without the least amount of concern. We know that there were many different causes of the paralysis of polio and that without massive amounts of ingested pesticides, no one is likely to have a problem. Even if we lived in a country where DDT or lead arsenate ingestion was a problem, we realize that the polio vaccine only protects from the poliovirus infection, but none of the several other viruses or bacteria that could also cause paralysis if given the same opportunity.

The narrow focus of the polio vaccine on the poliovirus, when many other microbes can also cause paralysis, actually represents a much bigger problem with vaccines—one that actually gives me comfort in skipping other shots for my family.

Chapter 16
The HIB Vaccine

Another vaccine that will be offered for your child at their 2-month checkup is the H.I.B. or Hib shot. HIB is an abbreviation of *Haemophilus Influenza Type B*. There are actually at least six different types of this bacteria, maybe more, but type B seems to be the one that can cause some problems, particularly with infants. Most people had never even heard of it before vaccines for this infection began to come out around 1987—it was that rare. Actually, the *infection* was common, but it rarely caused problems. In fact, most unvaccinated kids develop immunity to type B by the time they're five years old and their parents don't even realize it. For some reason, the most dangerous reaction to the infection, meningitis—when the lining of your brain becomes inflamed—is 4 times more common in black children.

Like pertussis, or whooping cough, this infection is only a concern during the first months of life—maybe a bit longer than whooping cough, like up to a year old. Thankfully, for healthy babies it's usually a trivial infection and is not considered very contagious. Your baby is probably a thousand times more likely to get injured in a car accident on the way to get this vaccine than being harmed by the infection it might prevent. Obviously, the bacteria can sometimes cause problems and for that reason, a vaccine was created to deal with this particular strain.

This vaccine creates a fairly weak immune response, and because of this, they'll want your child to get it multiple times during the first year of their life. With multiple doses of the Hib vaccine, it does appear to work fairly well at preventing this specific type of infection. Unfortunately, some of the versions of this vaccine contain aluminum, something I would never allow to be injected into me or my family. Many new parents don't know this, but most vaccines actually have several variations, manufactured differently by pharmaceutical companies. Some of the Hib vaccines don't contain aluminum. Some of them do contain a tiny amount of formaldehyde, but at such low quantities that even I wouldn't worry about it. It's really the aluminum I would look out for.

For me, the aluminum-containing versions of this vaccine would be a firm *no* for me. But what about the versions that don't contain aluminum? Would I want my infant to get this shot if it didn't contain aluminum? This is probably the one shot I might consider for my child but for a couple of things. One, the risk from the infection is so low. It really is minuscule—I'm not kidding about it being more dangerous to drive to the doctor's office to get the shot than the risk from this infection. Of course it would stink if your child did develop a problem from this infection and you felt like you could have done something that would have prevented it. That's why many parents vaccinate their kids for infections they wouldn't otherwise worry about—it's that fear of regret.

Something I haven't spoken about much yet is the injection itself. I'm like any other parent or kid—I hate injections. They just feel wrong. But I've done a bunch of research into them and there are two things I've got to mention real quick that make me reluctant to recommend any injections for my family unless they are completely necessary. One is polio. Yes, polio. They don't call it polio. They call it other things, but occasionally, viruses that are living on your skin can get pushed into your nervous system by an injection and cause paralysis. You've probably seen stories in the news recently of children coming down with mystery cases of "polio-like" paralysis? Some of these children were undoubtedly paralyzed by an injection. It wasn't an ingredient within a vaccine, but the physical injection itself that pierced the skin and pushed a virus into their nervous system. This is thankfully rare, and if you make sure the nurse is extra thorough with cleaning the skin with an alcohol swab and uses a clean needle, it should never happen. But unfortunately, it does happen, and knowing this happens makes me avoid injections for family if at all possible. I realize there are medical procedures that require injections like insulin shots and anesthesia for surgery. You can't avoid them all, but unless they're absolutely necessary, I would try to find a different way to protect my family.

The other issue I have with vaccines is the psychological effects. I have put a lot of effort into understanding why the aluminum in vaccines sometimes seems to target the brainstem. There is such a tiny amount of aluminum in these vaccines but sometimes a lot of it seems to go to the brain—and I wanted to know why. I'll talk more about it in the autism chapter, but the aluminum in vaccines gets picked up by your body's white blood cells because they think they're invaders. These white blood cells don't just float around your body randomly, but go where they're signaled to go.

Unfortunately, when you are very afraid, particularly if you are being immobilized or restrained, and you can't fight back or run away, your brainstem signals for help from your white blood cells.

We don't totally understand why this is, but if you are being pinned down and being stabbed with a needle, you can imagine your brain is going to actively signal for help from your white blood cells. If you happen to get injected with aluminum at this same time, that aluminum is not going to have much problem reaching your brain in this scenario.

I should tell you that this is a personal hypothesis of mine. The science is there to support it, but it's just a hypothesis. I don't know if it's true, and to be honest with you, I hope it's not true. Regardless, because of the psychological effects of immobilizing and restraining a child required for vaccines, I won't do it. One day there might be an epidemic of Ebola that's killing thousands and despite our best efforts we are unable to stop it. If there was a vaccine that appeared to have a chance at stopping it, I would consider it for my family. For the Hib vaccine, even though it actually appears to work fairly well, I would not want my child to have this shot.

Chapter 17
The Pneumococcal Vaccine

The *pneumococcal* vaccine will be recommended for your child at their 2-month checkup and beyond. It is designed to protect against a particular bacteria called *Streptococcus pneumoniae*, sometimes called *Pneumococcus*, or PC for short. It's a very common bacteria, especially because there are many different strains of it floating around at any given time. While most people get pneumococcus infections and deal with them just fine, they can occasionally cause problems for children or the elderly. The most tricky complication is *pneumonia*—when your lungs get inflamed and can build up with fluid.

This vaccine has to use aluminum as an ingredient, which means I would refuse it for my child, no matter what. But it has another big problem that most doctors or health officials won't mention to you. The original version of this vaccine protected against the 7 most common strains. As a lot of kids started to get this vaccine, other strains began to gain the upper hand. Those original 7 strains now account for only 2% of pneumococcus infections. Some of the new strains that emerged were resistant to antibiotics, making them more dangerous than the original seven. So a new vaccine was required and they made it—one that protected against 13 different strains of the bacteria. Fast-forward to today, and unfortunately, the same thing has happened again. New strains are emerging, ones which may be even *more* resistant to antibiotics than the original seven. There is another, slightly older version of the vaccine which covers 23 strains, but it isn't usually given to children unless they have a problem with their spleen or something similar.

This phenomenon begins to highlight what I consider a real problem when we start monkeying with nature in ways that we don't totally understand. You will see a similar problem when you read the chickenpox chapter, but I will say it time and again: Nothing is free. Everything has a cost. Not a financial cost, but when it comes to vaccines, a health cost. By creating a vaccine that minimized the effects of a few strains of the pneumococcus bacteria, we have created another problem. In slaying the 7-headed monster, we gave birth to a bigger, more powerful 13-headed monster. Who knows what problems we might create with this latest vaccine?

You should know that throughout history, diseases have always died natural deaths. They might flame up, seemingly out of nowhere, but each generation, they usually get weaker and weaker. This is how many vaccines are actually made—a microbe is grown over and over, hoping that it will eventually get weak enough to safely inject into someone. This is how the Plague—the Black Death that killed millions—disappeared. It eventually weakened to the point it wasn't able to sustain its killing spree. Should a vaccine have been invented for that?

Well we *now* know the bacteria was being spread by fleas on rats. We could probably easily control such an outbreak today—no vaccine necessary, no risk of inadvertently creating some other form of the germ that is even more destructive. If you spend any amount of time researching smallpox, you will probably come to the conclusion it also died a natural death, just like the Plague did. The smallpox vaccine worked very poorly, and there were never enough people globally to have eradicated it. Based on years of research, I don't believe we, as humans, have ever truly eradicated any diseases. Certainly not smallpox or polio—not with trillions and trillions of them floating in the air at any given time.

Look, there are certainly horrible diseases that scientists have every right to try and develop a vaccine for, but we just need to remember as human beings it will always come with a cost. The Hib vaccine actually has created this same problem—new strains have emerged which are more powerful than the original ones. One step forward, two steps back.

For this reason, and because the pneumococcal shot contains aluminum, I would not want my child to have this vaccine. I would focus on improving their health, nutrition, and happiness. I would recommend breast feeding as long as possible, well past their first birthday. I would try and reduce any sources of stress in their life. I would try to avoid daycare if possible. I realize this may not be realistic—but we all do what we can.

By now, you should realize that a focus on creating optimal health is probably the best protection against many of these infections you'll ever create. We will get these infections all the time, but with optimal health, they're unlikely to ever turn into serious problems. Best of all, there are no side effects.

Chapter 18
The Rotavirus Vaccine

Another vaccine your child will be recommended at their 2-month checkup is the *rotavirus* vaccine. Rotavirus is a common infection—it starts off like any common stomach bug but can cause a severe case of diarrhea. In first world countries, it is not considered a dangerous disease. The only real danger comes from your baby becoming dehydrated from days and days of diarrhea without offsetting it with liquids. Most anyone whose child has been having days of diarrhea is going to go see their doctor and take care of this problem but occasionally some people don't pay enough attention to realize their baby is getting dehydrated.

Rotavirus is spread by the pleasantly-named *fecal-oral* route. Basically, if your child is around places like the changing table at your local daycare, the chance of them getting this virus goes way up. Regardless, it is so common it may be impossible to avoid. As an adult, you most likely already have immunity to rotavirus and if you are breastfeeding your infant and passing on your immunity to them, the likelihood of your child developing aggressive diarrhea from an infection is small.

Like some forms of the polio vaccine, the rotavirus vaccine employs drops administered by mouth. Occasionally your infant may spit them out and your doctor may not be sure if they swallowed it, but the fact it is *not* an injection is encouraging to me—someone who hates injections. It also doesn't contain aluminum—another huge plus in my book. Unfortunately, there are two other problems that would prevent me from accepting this vaccine for my child.

One is a strange side effect called *intussusception*. Intussusception is when your intestine kind of folds over itself like a telescope tube. Doctors are not really sure why this happens but for some reason, both of the rotavirus vaccines seem to increase the risk of intussusception. This dramatic event can cause intestinal blockages and death if left untreated, and in third-world countries, something like this will often go untreated. For the unlikely chance my child develops some aggressive diarrhea, I wouldn't risk the unlikely chance they develop intussusception. No one wants surgery for their infant so I'd choose aggressive hydration over surgery any day.

Another problem with this vaccine is that it's produced from the organs of other animals—namely pigs and baboons. Way back in the 1950s, it was discovered that the polio vaccine contained at least 40 different viruses—microbes that were being transferred from the monkey tissue the vaccines were being grown in. One of them was known to cause cancer in humans, a concerning anecdote because the AIDS virus was another monkey virus that somehow migrated into human beings where it has obviously caused serious problems.

Many other vaccines are grown in animal tissue, but the pig and baboon DNA that would inevitably be ingested by my child from this vaccine gives me a bit of concern. Many vaccines are produced using animal tissue—the flu shot is grown in chicken eggs if you didn't already know. There is something about the possibility of pig or baboon DNA getting into my child that really bothers me. I don't think they're going to turn into animals but because the vaccine isn't injected, but taken orally by mouth, I'm not going to obsess over it. Injected is always 100 times worse than ingested.

The final issue with this vaccine is it seems to cause other gastrointestinal problems not related to the rotavirus. It is a live vaccine, which can occasionally cause an actual rotavirus infection. While that is a problem, something else occasionally comes up. For reasons we don't understand, a lot of kids seem to develop other stomach and intestinal issues after taking this vaccine. It may have reduced the chance of a rotavirus infection while creating another problem in the process.

If you live in a first world country, the danger of this infection is minimal. If you're breastfeeding your baby, it's even less likely something bad will happen. If your child isn't hanging around the changing table at a nursery, they will probably not even get an infection until later in their life, when you can more easily keep them hydrated. Because the only serious danger from a rotavirus infection is dehydration—something easily avoided—and the risk of intussusception is there, I would never recommend this vaccine for my own family.

Chapter 19
The Vaccine Schedule

I want to talk to you about the vaccine schedule your doctor's office is going to recommend your child adhere to. You may think the vaccine schedule is a universally accepted set of shots children all around the world receive, if they're able, but the truth is, this schedule differs wildly based on which country you are in.

You may think the schedule varies between countries based on which diseases they tend to struggle with, but that is not always the case. Those who set public health policy regarding vaccination typically have the opposite mindset of someone like me. I want as few vaccines as possible, while they see no limit to the amount of vaccines a child might receive—the more, the better. I prefer improving their health naturally to make it easier to fight off infection, while they would prefer your children rely on pharmaceutical interventions.

In the United States, we have the most aggressive vaccination schedule by far. For a country with better medical care, hygiene, and nutrition than most countries, it might seem odd that we vaccinate for so many diseases—and it is. It *is* odd. Many European countries have a similar mindset to me—they err on the side of caution and only recommend a vaccine if they feel it is absolutely necessary.

For instance, most European countries don't recommend the hepatitis B vaccine at all. They might suggest the mother be tested for hepatitis B and then make a decision, but even so, they would never imagine injecting a one-hour-old infant with a vaccine of any type. In the United States, it is strongly recommended no matter what—even if you test negative for hepatitis B and there is essentially zero risk for your baby, they will strongly recommend that shot. Why? Because it's on the vaccine schedule, that's why! Most doctors and nurses have not studied the cost vs. benefit of various vaccines—they simply take the schedule at face value.

Many European countries don't recommend children get the chickenpox shot—also called the *varicella* vaccine—your child will be offered at their one-year well-child visit. In the Netherlands, they don't even ask school children to stay home. Chickenpox is a rite of passage, a trivial infection every kid gets and if other kids pick it up from them, they aren't concerned. They even have chickenpox songs they sing in class whenever children get the infection. In the U.S., the news will report on chickenpox infections as if the world is about to end. Strange isn't it? Why are some countries so afraid when others have no fear at all?

In the U.S., where many vaccine manufacturers are based, they work very hard with government health officials to maximize the fear of disease they make vaccines for. This may seem like an outlandish statement, but you can easily find Powerpoint presentations from their strategy meetings and you will see how this is one of their main strategic goals—to create fear. Before the chickenpox vaccine came along, no one was dying from chickenpox. No one was begging for a chickenpox vaccine—they made it because scientific discovery had progressed to the point where they could.

Once the vaccine came out, efforts to make chickenpox infections—an event for which kindergarteners sing songs about in other countries—into campaigns of fear began. It's a crazy concept that is difficult to accept is actually happening. To believe this means that people in charge of our children's health may be less than honest with us. They may be trying to manipulate us for some personal gain. I don't think most in power are doing this for financial reasons—I think they truly believe they're making the world a healthier place for children and they're willing to act a little less ethically if that's what it takes. Many corporations obviously benefit from these actions, but the source of it is not some evil conspiracy starving for more money, just other good-natured people who want what's best for children. Good intentions, but the result can be very different than what was intended.

Japan has a much different vaccine schedule than Europeans, as do many other countries. Because of daily international travel, the ability for a virus or bacteria to move from any part of the world to another makes the quarantine of infection nearly impossible. Every country may face a potential infection every day from anywhere on the planet. The vaccine schedules differ because some country's health officials can apply more political pressure to add more shots than others. In the U.S., the pharmaceutical lobby is the most well-financed political pressure cooker in the world. Because of this, they have been successful in essentially forcing many vaccines on children that parents (and their doctors) never asked for.

I would take a look at some of the other countries vaccine schedules and realize that the shots being recommended to your children often are there not because of an urgent risk of harm from an infection, but simply because of the immense political pressure the pharmaceutical lobby is able to apply.

Chapter 20
The 4-Month Checkup

Once your baby has reached their 4-month mark, doctors recommend you head into their office for another appointment. Like the 2-month checkup, they'll measure your baby's length, weight and head circumference. They may check for some basic reflexes, but the real reason you are there is for more shots—basically a repeat of the shots they had been offered two months earlier. For vaccines that were originally supposed to work forever, but now are advertised as working for a few years, possibly less, it should seem odd they feel like the eight vaccines your child just received two months earlier are in danger of not working.

The reality is that many vaccines don't work so good. Some kids just don't develop a very strong immune response and we're not sure why. To make sure their immune system got the message, doctors will ask to inject your kids again a few more times—like at this 4-month appointment where your child might receive those same eight vaccines again: One for rotavirus, polio, diphtheria, tetanus, pertussis, pneumonia, hepatitis B, and HiB. It doesn't matter whether the original ones worked perfectly, your child will be asked to get most of these four more times. By now, the one illness that I'd be concerned about—pertussis, or whooping cough—should be much less of a danger. Your baby should have begun to develop enough muscle tone in their stomach and diaphragm to cough properly. If they were to happen to catch a pertussis infection, they should be able to cough the mucus from their lungs and not develop any problems.

If you really wanted to know if additional vaccines were necessary, you could do titer tests for each infection, which check for the presence of antibodies in your child's blood and provide a partial view into whether the vaccine worked or not. Some veterinarians do this before administering additional rabies shots. They'll test your dog's rabies titers and just skip additional shots if it appears your dog is already immune. Because my goal is to administer as few vaccines as possible to my child, and if I had already given them all the vaccines from the 2-month well-child visit, I would absolutely skip these. The effect of multiple versions of the same vaccine appears to decrease each time. The antibodies may go up for a month or so, but come back down to where they were after the first shot. And after each additional shot, they come back down even quicker (and don't go up as high). This is part of the reason why they make "increased dosage" flu shots for the elderly. They're discovering after years and years of flu shots, they begin to respond really poorly to each year's vaccine, no matter which strain the shot was manufactured from.

If you really wanted your child to have those original vaccines, just know that each additional vaccine appears to work less and less. If my child already had those first few shots and they were due for the next round soon, I would skip them. If they worked, they worked. If they didn't, they didn't. I wouldn't risk any additional harm to my children from any of the aluminum-containing vaccines for what is likely to be a decreasing response from their immune system. You might want to save it in case they travel, later on in their life. Maybe a vaccine right before they leave would give them enough of a boost to help them, but probably not if they'd had five or six of the shots already—the boosting effect appears to be eventually lost.

So as you approach your 4-month visit, just know these are a repeat of the 2-month shots—just in case they didn't work. For someone who is trying for as few vaccines as possible, I would never double up, triple up, or quadruple up, just in case they didn't work the first time. I'd want to know for sure they didn't work before I administered them again.

Chapter 21
The Flu/Influenza Vaccine

At your baby's 6-month well-child visit, your doctor is likely to recommend a new vaccine if they haven't already offered it—the flu shot. The flu shot is probably one of the most commonly mentioned —and commonly skipped—vaccines in the United States, if not other countries. You've no doubt heard of many people saying they caught the flu after getting the flu shot and other problems with the vaccine. Other reports will talk about whether they "guessed the right strain" this year or not. If they guess the right strain, then the shot works better. If not, it doesn't work so good.

I want to give you the truth about the flu shot, because you really need to know it now, before you ever give your child their first influenza vaccine. There are 3 different types of influenza virus which can cause the symptoms we call the flu. If you haven't had the flu recently, I will refresh your memory—it is horrible. I had it once as a kid but hadn't had it since until a few years ago. I felt like death for about two days as I battled through a flu infection. I had no recollection of it being that bad, but it was horrible. I felt cold. I felt hot. I was shivering and burning up at the same time. I would hate for my child to have to go through that—I really would.

As we all know, the flu shot has problems—serious problems. It has never worked very well, and they've been trying to perfect it for decades, since the 1940s. You will hear that "guessing the right strain" phrase over and over, but the truth about things is much more complex. The influenza virus doesn't have an offseason, where it takes a break and morphs into something else, like a butterfly emerging from a cocoon. It is constantly mutating—all the time. Sometimes it's little changes, other times big changes. We have no idea from year to year what strains are going to be prevalent, and we don't have any idea how quickly and in what directions they will mutate.

Because of this, the influenza vaccine is like trying to hit a moving target. The microbes don't just change once a year, but all the time, every day, every hour. Sometimes they change less, and if manufacturers guessed the right strain, the shot might work a little better. Often times, the virus changes enough that the vaccine just doesn't work. You might hear them say the flu shot is 19% effective this year—as if that's a good thing. A respectable science foundation figured out that on average 71 people had to get the flu shot for it to protect one person from getting the flu. The other 70 people it didn't work for. This is so pitiful, I can't believe health officials and doctors will go on TV acting serious about people getting their flu shot. It is such a horrible product the manufacturers would be sued out of existence if it were any industry. Imagine buying some 71 bottles of formula for your baby and realizing that only one of them actually contained something helpful, while the others made him sick. That wouldn't go over very well anywhere outside of the pharmaceutical industry. For some reason, when it's vaccines—we just accept it. It's very strange.

Another thing you'll hear over and over again is that even if the flu shot didn't prevent you from getting the flu, it might have prevented it from being worse. This is false and unscientifically supported. If you ask a doctor or nurse to show you the science that supports this, they'll come up empty. Vaccines are designed for specific strains of viruses or bacteria. This is *why* the 7-strain pneumococcal vaccine was changed to the 13-strain. The original 7-strain shot did nothing for the other strains other than make them grow stronger. The original HPV Gardasil vaccine was replaced by a newer one that fought more strains. In fact, the science suggests that you are more likely to get an infection from another strain by getting the flu shot. This is why you'll often hear people say the flu shot gave them the flu. The flu shot doesn't have the ability to actually give them the flu, like a live-virus vaccine might, but it will suppress your immune system so much that it makes you much more susceptible to getting an infection from another strain of the influenza virus.

This is why children have a higher rate of respiratory infections after getting the flu shot. It may boost your immunity for a very specific thing, but it comes at a cost—you lose a bit of immunity somewhere else as your body fights the invader the vaccine introduced. We are just now beginning to realize how much we *don't* understand about this. They call it *non-specific effects* and it's really scary. When they develop vaccines, of course they look for and measure the effect the shot is supposed to produce. But what we are now realizing is that vaccines don't just produce that specific effect, but often produce many other effects that they were never even looking for.

The last thing I want to talk about also applies to other vaccines, but particularly this one. The effectiveness of the flu shot appears to be reduced the more often you get it. Let me put it another way—repeated annual flu shots make them work less. If you haven't had a flu shot in five years, this year's might work okay. If you had one the year before, and the year before that, this year's shot may be completely useless. Like the non-specific effects I was just talking about, we don't understand why this is. But you do see it in other vaccines. As people get older, and they've had a ton of flu shots, they become more and more susceptible to other infections—possibly the flu itself most of all.

I could go on and on about the ridiculousness of the flu shot, but I won't. I want to tell you something you may have a hard time believing. The numbers of people that die from the flu every year are greatly exaggerated. Many of these people are sickly or elderly people who died from pneumonia or some other complication. If their death can be even remotely attributed to the flu, they'll usually get assigned to that column. Why? Those people who profit from and whose professions rely on promoting vaccines subconsciously know that fear sells. So because the annual flu shot is their biggest product (every person on the planet, once a year), they really want to make sure the fear of the flu is constantly front and center in everyone's mind. If you're an older person, or have some other illness, I would be concerned about getting the flu and would exercise caution during the winter months by keeping my hands washed and avoiding crowded, enclosed spaces. Most of all, I would avoid the flu shot like the plague. Knowing that it suppresses your immune system in ways we don't totally understand, I would avoid it completely.

If it were my child, I would never let them have the flu shot. There is no way I would wreck their immune system, year after year, like that. I would hate it if they got the flu. It's miserable. But knowing in their natural state they're much better off fighting that and other infections long-term gives me confidence that when it comes to influenza, natural immunity is definitely the way to go.

Chapter 22
The 9-Month Checkup

The 9-month checkup is very similar to previous checkups. Measurements, reflex tests, and a chance to ask your doctor questions about any concerns you have. By now, you will have realized the reason these visits exist are to administer shots, and not much more. Depending on how your previous well-child visits went, and which—if any—vaccines were administered, your doctor may have catch-up shots already waiting for your son or daughter.

Taking your healthy baby to a pediatric office full of sick kids is not something anyone wants to do, and just like how I try to minimize the number of vaccines administered to my family, I would also minimize the number of doctor visits. Depending on your insurance situation, it may not be a financial concern at all. Regardless, doctor's offices are typically full of sick people and to purposefully expose your family and yourself to these germs without good reason may not be worth it. Some doctors have separate waiting rooms for sick and healthy children, but often share the same bathrooms, door knobs, and air handlers. I've heard of some extra cautious doctors who schedule healthy well-child visits in the morning and reserve the afternoon for sick patients. This may offer enough separation to prevent a rogue infection from happening.

If it were me, unless I had a true concern about my child—like an ongoing infection that wouldn't clear up, or some behavioral or possibly neurological event, like changes in their facial symmetry or feeding patterns—I wouldn't go to a single well-child visit unless there was a specific vaccine I wanted my child to receive. There is really no other reason for these visits. You may feel, as a new mother, these appointments to be a safety net of support. They can give you confidence you are doing a good job and that your baby is doing fine. The reality is, your maternal instinct is the most finely-tuned problem detector on the planet. Unfortunately, our medical establishment has made many young ladies into terrified, petrified mothers, but if there is anything other mothers would tell you, it is to trust yourself. Listen to your inner voice. Learn to hear it. It's been drowned out by a million rules about this and that, and many of us don't live close enough to our families to have our own mothers lend us a hand. Don't worry about any of that. You could probably harm your baby less on purpose than a careless physician could do on accident. If something feels wrong, say something. See your doctor. If everything feels okay, enjoy it. Celebrate it. Don't feel like you have to go to a well-child visit just to check off a box somewhere. Unless you have a true concern, their only purpose is to administer vaccines to your child, and almost nothing else.

By the time your 2nd or 3rd child comes around, they may not even have been to a doctor's office until many years later, even in to their teens. I'd count this as a blessing and a sign of good health. Like creating a baby, and having a baby, raising a baby is not a medical emergency by default. It should be a beautiful experience free of trauma if possible. For me, and for my family, I want as few vaccines as possible. And as few doctor visits as possible. For those with infants, those usually go hand in hand.

Chapter 23
The Measles Vaccine

At your baby's 12-month well-child visit, in addition to many of the other vaccines they may have already given your baby 3 doses of, they will have a few new ones to add—measles, mumps, rubella, and hepatitis A. I want to talk about measles for now. Measles is an infection most people have heard of, but if you're a younger parent, you're unlikely to have ever seen it. I'm a little bit older, and when I was growing up, the measles vaccine wasn't that popular, so it was common for my classmates to get measles and stay home from school for a few days.

In first world countries, measles was considered a trivial infection before the vaccine came out for it. There is a famous Brady Bunch episode where all the kids get measles. No one is scared in the least—it's treated as a joke. The kids are actually excited because they get to stay home from school and play games. This episode aired in 1967, before the measles vaccine became popular. Now that we have a vaccine, people are terrified of it. So strange how a trivial infection becomes scary once a vaccine is made for it. Fear is a powerful marketing tool. People are very rich because of it.

Measles is a viral infection that often produces red bumps on your body. There are many other infections that can create similar effects, so it can actually be difficult just by looking to tell if your child has measles. It has all of the same symptoms of a typical fever —runny nose, cough, and not feeling very good, and of course, the red dots. There is a very rare side effect of measles which can cause *encephalitis*—which is swelling of the brain. In first world countries, where nutrition is usually good, complications from measles are *extremely* rare—almost non-existent. They discovered that vitamin A deficiency has a way of making measles infections worse and is usually the reason you hear of children dying of measles in third world countries. If you live in a first world country or your child is not malnourished, I would watch the Brady Bunch episode and realize they had no fear of the infection before the vaccine. There is no reason to fear it now.

What about the measles vaccine? People have a lot of questions about it because in the United States, it comes as part of a combo shot with mumps and rubella vaccines. It's called the MMR shot— for measles, mumps and rubella. You can't get them separately—at least in the U.S. The MMR has a bit of a nasty reputation because many parents who have said their children developed autism after vaccination often point to the MMR shot as the trigger. There were a few studies that looked at the association between the mercury preservative some of these shots used to contain and autism, but as far as I know, never the shot itself (and certainly not other shots or their ingredients like aluminum, the one I'm really concerned with).

The MMR shot doesn't currently contain aluminum or mercury, yet it is still associated with autism and other neurological problems. Why is this? I have a hypothesis as to why I believe this happens but it's fairly complex. I explain it thoroughly in another book of mine called *The Autism Vaccine* but if you like, you can read the chapter on autism in this book where I do my best to explain it simply. Without going into much detail at this point, I believe the measles component is the problem with these neurological issues parents sometimes see after the MMR shot. It used to contain mercury, and people thought that was the problem. It may have contributed to it, but I don't think that was actually the problem.

Even though the MMR vaccine doesn't contain aluminum (or mercury), I would not recommend it for my child. The risk of complications from a measles infection is extremely low and the long-term protection it provides is not very good. It may give you a temporary boost in measles-fighting antibodies, but the lifelong immunity they want it to provide usually only lasts a few years, sometimes as few as two or three. If you're thinking, "Doesn't that mean that most everyone walking around who is older than 10 years old is probably vulnerable to a measles infection?" then you are correct. Most anyone who hasn't had an MMR shot in the past few years is vulnerable to a measles infection. Older people, most of whom probably got a measles infection naturally, don't have to worry. They are immune for life, and in fact, many places will accept your proof of age as a sign you have measles immunity (they trust that more than a shot). Strange but true.

Just in case you didn't notice it in any of the other chapters, nine months is the age at which I really become concerned about administering vaccines—mainly because of the psychological impact of these procedures. At 3, 6, or 9 months your baby probably has no idea what's coming—all they know is something really painful has stung their arm or legs. At 12 months, and especially at 15 and 18 months, the fear factor really begins to elevate. As a result, the amount of physical force required to restrain or immobilize your kid to be able to safely administer shots to them also goes up. I believe this is a very bad thing to do in combination with aluminum or live-virus containing vaccines. I talk about it more in the autism chapter, but if there were a vaccine I felt compelled to administer to my child, I would do everything possible to wait until they weren't afraid of it—until they could understand that it was supposed to help them. If it requires physical restraint or immobilization, I wouldn't do it. Not because I'm afraid they'll hate me, but because of the immunological sequence of events it can create.

Chapter 24
The Mumps Vaccine

Mumps is the other "M" in the MMR vaccine—another vaccine your child will be offered at their 1-year check up. I'll go ahead and say that I'm not a big fan of the MMR vaccine because of it's association with neurological side-effects. I believe this is mostly due to the measles component of the vaccine, but I want to talk about mumps so you can understand this infection and decide whether it's something you're afraid of or not.

Mumps is a viral infection whose most distinguishing characteristic is it tends to infect the salivary glands right in front of your ears, causing your cheeks or neck to look like they're puffed up. For some reason, mumps almost never causes any problems in children. It is completely harmless almost *all* the time. It is only teens and adults that can develop issues, sometimes with their reproductive organs. Brain swelling can be a complication, but thankfully even in teens and adults, this is completely rare—no matter the country you live in. If you get a mumps infection as a child, as everyone used to do, you would be immune for life and you would never have to worry about it later on when it might be a bit more dangerous. Now that we have a vaccine for mumps that provides a kind of half-protection that only lasts for a few years, you see outbreaks happen on college campuses now and then. This would've never happened before the vaccine because all of those kids would've received lifelong protection from a natural infection. Now, we depend on boosters to keep us safe. Not an improvement, in my opinion.

I'm not really sure why the mumps vaccine was even manufactured. It was an innocuous infection that no one really cared about. Kids weren't dying or becoming handicapped from mumps infections. It was just a simple infection like chickenpox or measles that every kid was expected to get at some point. But a vaccine was made, and like all other diseases, once a vaccine has been made, we become terrified of the disease.

Because the mumps vaccine is not available separately, you will either get the vaccine or not depending on your choice about the MMR shot. As I said in the previous chapter, because mumps is such a trivial infection that rarely causes problems, and because the vaccine itself is associated with neurological side effects—rare though they might be—I would skip the mumps vaccine for my child without the least bit of fear. In fact, this is one of those infections like chickenpox I would prefer my child get naturally at a young age, when it appears to be most safe.

Chapter 25
The Rubella Vaccine

Another vaccine you child will be recommended at their 1-year checkup is for rubella. Rubella is typically the "R" in the MMR vaccine, although it may be available in some places as a single shot. Measles, mumps and rubella. Rubella is occasionally called *German measles* because it looks so similar to regular old measles. It is another mild infection and often doesn't even cause red spots to appear. Most people who got a rubella infection naturally don't even realize they got it. The only reason a vaccine exists for rubella is because if you are pregnant and get rubella it can cause a birth defect. This was an extremely rare event, but occasionally a girl would make it through her childhood without catching rubella, only to catch it while she was in the first trimester of her pregnancy.

Because of this, a vaccine was created for rubella and it was lumped in alongside the measles and mumps vaccines. You can't make a choice whether you get just the rubella vaccine in the U.S., but if it were me, I would skip it—not only because of the reasons I mentioned in the measles and mumps chapters (trivial infection, side effects from the vaccine), but also something else. If it works properly, the vaccine only protects you for a few years but remember, pregnancy in females is the thing we're concerned with. Out of the whole MMR vaccine, rubella is actually the only component that I feel *might* be worthwhile. Obviously, anyone would hate for their daughter to have a child with birth defects. But the shot doesn't work for more than a few years, so to give an infant girl the rubella shot in hopes of protecting her while she is pregnant is pointless. Completely meaningless.

If I had a son, and because autism is so much more prevalent with boys, I would definitely avoid the MMR shot completely. If I had a daughter, I might one day try to find a way to get a standalone rubella vaccine—if it were available—but giving it to her 15 years before she might have children is a complete waste. A needless risk. If you get lucky, she'll get the infection naturally as a child and she'll never have to worry about it. As I mentioned earlier, the problem is most people don't even realize they got it. You'd have to do a test to see if you have immunity to it. Regardless, rubella is so rare these days, even a pregnant woman is unlikely to have to worry about it.

Chapter 26
The Chickenpox/Varicella Vaccine

Let's talk about the chickenpox vaccine, otherwise known as the *Varicella* shot. At your 1-year checkup, they will suggest your child receive this shot. The *Varicella zoster* virus causes chickenpox, a very mild infection not known for creating any problems other than a bunch of little red itchy pocks all over your body. This is a live virus vaccine, meaning it does occasionally have the ability to mutate into the actual infection, but even the actual infection isn't a concern. Varicella is a relatively new vaccine—it was first introduced in 1995, so if you were born around or before then, you might have not received it.

Because chickenpox is so mild, many other countries don't even offer a vaccine for it. In fact, some countries don't even send children home for school with it—even though it's contagious. Why? Are public health officials completely crazy? Actually, no. Chickenpox used to be considered a trivial infection in the U.S. before a vaccine was introduced for it. People had neighborhood parties for their children to purposefully get infected. It was considered a rite of passage for childhood, and because it seems to be a bit more dangerous for adults, most people wanted their children to get the infection over with so they would never have to worry about it again.

In the Netherlands, schools are so unconcerned with the infection they even have chickenpox songs they sing in class during an outbreak. "One pox here, two pox there," and so on as they point to the red dots on their faces or shoulders. They literally treat chickenpox as if a swarm of ladybugs had invaded their classroom and landed on some of the students. In the U.S., we used to treat the infection the same way. No one was afraid of it, and no one, especially parents, was begging for a chickenpox vaccine. But in 1995, pharmaceutical companies were successful in getting their new chickenpox shot added to the childhood vaccine schedule—not because children were dying from the infection, but because it would make them a lot of money. Ever since the vaccine was added to the schedule, chickenpox has become a scary disease. It really makes it clear how ignorant people are about infections and vaccines when you just take a look at how other countries whose health programs aren't controlled by the pharmaceutical lobby treat certain infections.

And in another twist of good intentions gone wrong, the aggressive vaccination of children for the varicella zoster virus created another problem—an explosion of *shingles* in the elderly population. Shingles is an extremely painful rash that is caused by a latent infection of varicella zoster virus. It used to be a rare event, but ever since they started vaccinating children for chickenpox, the incidence of shingles has exploded. Scientists believe this explosion may be because in the time before the chickenpox vaccine, the elderly were frequently exposed to children with chickenpox infections. This effect—called *exogenous boosting*—acted like a natural immune boosting agent and was able to keep shingles outbreaks away. Now that we've monkeyed with things, shingles has exploded. And believe me, it's painful—I got it a few years ago and can vouch for the descriptions of it. Now the same company that created the chickenpox vaccine has a shingles vaccine to take care of the problem caused by the first vaccine. Science to the rescue!

Because chickenpox is such a trivial infection that other schools sing songs about, and because the absence of natural chickenpox infections have caused an explosion in shingles, I would never let my child have this vaccine. You and your children's grandparents will thank you one day.

Chapter 27
The Hepatitis A Vaccine

Hepatitis A is an extremely rare viral infection that can negatively affect your liver's ability to function. When someone does get a hepatitis A infection, it's usually through contaminated food. You may recall an occasional news story about a restaurant temporarily shutting down for a few days as they sterilize the whole place? This is probably due to someone having come down with a hepatitis A infection after having eaten there. In adults, the infection can cause extreme fatigue, joint pains, nausea, vomiting, and many other unpleasant side effects. For some reason, in children the infection seems to be completely mild. In fact, many children get the infection without their parents even noticing.

The hepatitis A vaccine was not made with children in mind, but for some reason, the CDC began recommending that children get it in 2006. For a disease this rare and completely trivial, it boggles my mind why the CDC would have made the recommendation that all children receive this vaccine. Remember that we're trying to create a healthy environment for our families to ensure they need the fewest vaccines possible. The CDC, on the other hand, seems like they would prefer your children receive as many vaccines as possible. I sometimes wonder if there are *any* number of vaccines they might consider too many for children. It's really disgusting to me how readily and happily they just recommend new vaccines for children with little concern as to the psychological effects of being injected another two or three or *seventy* times.

In addition to it not being necessary, the hepatitis A vaccine contains aluminum, a neurotoxin I would never allow my family to be injected with unless there was a life-threatening emergency. Thankfully, many states have not followed the CDC's recommendation and have not added the hepatitis A vaccine to their list of shots required for public school. You will have to check your states specific requirements if attending public school is in your children's future, especially if you live in California, West Virginia, Mississippi, or New York.

Because it contains aluminum, and because it is normally a completely rare, trivial infection in children, I would never allow my child to have this shot, under any circumstances. Like the other ridiculous childhood vaccine, hepatitis B, I would skip this shot with absolutely zero anxiety or fear.

Chapter 28
The Disease You Should Fear Most

Ask yourself something: What's the disease you fear most for your child? Without going on the internet and doing a search, what springs to mind? Think of the one disease you dread your child getting. Most people will say polio. Others may say whooping cough.

Think about this for a second—can you name a disease you are afraid of that doesn't have a vaccine? It's difficult for most. You may say Ebola or Zika, but most people can't name a disease they're afraid of that doesn't sit on the vaccine schedule. Why is this?

It's a strange phenomenon, but many people only fear the diseases listed on the childhood vaccine schedule. Do you fear tuberculosis? It's estimated to kill 1.7 million people each year. There *is* a vaccine for it. You could go get your child vaccinated for tuberculosis right now—a disease that kills millions of people each year—yet hardly anyone in the U.S. gets the vaccine or is afraid of tuberculosis. Why is that? Because it's *not* on the childhood vaccine schedule.

Think about measles. Measles was considered a trivial disease— even joked about on television shows. Decades later, now that a vaccine has been developed for it and is recommended for every child born in this country, public health officials and news media outlets lose their collective minds when someone comes down with a case of measles. Measles is much less dangerous than tuberculosis, but despite having vaccines for both of them, health officials and media reporters only seem to care about the one on the childhood schedule.

Chickenpox is the same way. A popular news show from the Netherlands recently featured a segment about picture day at the local kindergarten. This picture day was thought to be especially cute because nearly every child had chickenpox—their faces covered in dots. The photographer and teacher all came in to school, each child smiling for the camera, as if nothing was wrong.

Meanwhile, in the United States, where the vaccine is strongly suggested, news outlets cover a single chickenpox infection like it was a mass shooting. Children might be kept from school for weeks, despite the fact everyone is supposed to be protected from infection by the vaccine. In the Netherlands, the chickenpox shot is not recommended, and they treat an outbreak as a humorous, even joyful, story. In the U.S., the vaccine is strongly recommended and stories of the corresponding disease outbreak are treated as ominous threats to public health.

I'm not suggesting there is some kind of secret conspiracy to make you fear the diseases we have vaccines for, but when you see the pattern over and over again, it does begin to make you wonder. Why should we fear diseases we have vaccines for—shouldn't it be the opposite? Shouldn't we fear the diseases we don't have vaccines for?

The unfortunate reality behind this phenomenon is most parents don't like vaccines. Most kids don't like vaccines. This is understandable. They're painful injections that often make your arm hurt and possibly feel sick. But there is an underlying fear that goes beyond temporary pain. For many parents, vaccines just feel wrong. There is something unnatural about restraining a screaming child against their will and allowing someone to inject foreign material into their body.

If parents didn't have a lot of fear regarding these diseases, many would just skip the shots. So public health officials and the media work overtime to create and maintain fear of the diseases we have vaccines for—just to make sure you don't skip any. You will notice, that besides Ebola and Zika, they rarely spend time reporting about diseases for which there are no vaccines (Ebola and Zika vaccines may be licensed any day now).

Some health officials will admit that a bit of fear-mongering is necessary because the vaccines made us forget how bad the diseases actually were. This is clearly not the case with the hepatitis B or chickenpox shots and many other diseases weren't feared before vaccines were invented for them. If anything, we fear these particular diseases more now than we did before their vaccines—largely due to the scary stories the media produce to create fear. This fear begins to feel strange when you see how other countries respond to outbreaks of some of these diseases—look up the Netherlands chickenpox outbreak when you have a moment. Watch how they laugh about it.

This may seem like a strange phenomenon unconnected to your opinions about vaccines, but for me, it actually plays a very important role in my goal of as few vaccines as possible. If you would have asked me years ago what the one disease I feared my child getting, it would have been polio. Once I realized the likelihood of my child getting paralyzed was nearly zero because we don't coat their food in DDT or lead arsenate pesticides anymore, I felt completely confident in skipping the polio vaccine.

If you took polio off the list, I'm not really sure what I would have mentioned next. Nothing would have come to my mind—I would have to look over the childhood vaccine schedule and picked something. You may be afraid of the diseases we have vaccines for, but here's a very important thing to remember: there are thousands and thousands of other viruses and bacteria which could harm your children just as easily. We have vaccines for just a tiny percentage of known viruses and bacteria—probably less than .01%, yet you could probably not name a single one. You are afraid of the ones listed on the childhood vaccine schedule, but not the others.

If a child were to be harmed by one of these other viruses or bacteria, it would be unlikely to make the news because there is no vaccine for it. If it were a "vaccine-preventable disease," then it would be talked about for days on end. People like me recognize this phenomenon and realize that even if our children received every vaccine available on the planet (even more than the 72 recommended by U.S. health officials), it would still only protect them from a tiny fraction of the hundreds of thousands of varieties of microbes they might encounter any given day.

Instead of subjecting our children to potentially hundreds of injections, we focus on creating optimum health and nutrition. We believe that vaccines can interfere with proper immune system function and know that when optimum health and nutrition are present, the immune system can take care of nearly any infection—even the ones for which vaccines don't exist.

Chapter 29
How Natural Immunity Can Be Better

Although many of the vaccines on the childhood schedule could easily be considered unnecessary because the infection no longer poses a threat, many people like me might choose to skip some of them for another reason: vaccines screw up your immune system. This may come as a surprise to you, but our attempts to hijack the immune system with vaccines tend to create unintended consequences.

Most people think of vaccines as simply taking a harmful virus or bacteria, killing—or weakening it—so that it can't harm, and introducing it into the body to create an immune response without all the danger of getting the actual disease. Many vaccines don't actually work this way.

Take the pertussis, or whooping cough vaccine, for example. The pertussis vaccine—the "aP" in the DTaP vaccine—presents a really interesting example of how vaccines are inferior to natural infection. During a pertussis infection, the bacteria triggers the release of several toxins. One of them is extremely clever and is called *ACT*. ACT tricks your immune system into thinking nothing is wrong for about 14 days. This gives the infection a two-week head start before your immune system figures out what's really going on. During that time, the infection has time to get a solid foothold.

Eventually your immune system catches on and is able to develop protection against the ACT toxin. That's a good thing, because the next time you get a pertussis infection, your body will be prepared and the ACT sneak attack won't work. The next time you get an infection, it can be cleared easily because that two-week grace period will be gone.

When you receive a pertussis vaccine, your body's immune system gets programmed incorrectly. The pertussis vaccine doesn't protect against the ACT toxin—because they haven't figured out how to include that yet—so the vaccine forces your immune system to react to a pertussis infection differently than a natural infection. How? It reacts much more slowly.

Unfortunately, your body will never learn the 14-day ACT trick once you receive a pertussis vaccine. Even if you get a pertussis infection after you were vaccinated for it, your immune system has already been programmed incorrectly from the vaccine and can't be taught the correct way—ever! It can't un-learn the old way. This is why it's so important to have the correct immune response the first time. You basically get one chance to get things right. I'm oversimplifying this a bit, but the crucial component of the natural immune response to whooping cough is your body's ability to quickly recognize that specific toxin, ACT, and start mounting a defense. The vaccine specifically prevents your body from doing this.

Another interesting thing about ACT—you may have heard that many whooping cough outbreaks happening around the country actually might come from a different strain of bacteria than the one targeted in the vaccine—what they call *bordetella parapertussis*. This new strain may have been created because of the vaccine, kind of like how antibiotics can create this same problem.

The ACT trick is *also* used by the new strain of pertussis bacteria to get a two week head start on your immune system. If you had a natural pertussis infection, you will have developed ACT immunity correctly and would be able to fight off both infections, even though you were never vaccinated for bordetella parapertussis (because a vaccine doesn't exist for it). Nature is amazing like that.

Every vaccine is different, but nearly all of them have one or more problems like this. Nothing in life is free, and by trying to cheat mother nature's most complex invention—the immune system—we nearly always get something we didn't ask for. You may have seen recently how certain viruses like measles and polio are actually being used for cancer treatments? This just goes to show you how complex the interactions between the body and microbes can be.

Because we don't fully understand what kinds of problems vaccines may be creating with our immune system, and because these problems typically last forever, many parents are opting out of certain vaccines rather than risk permanently screwing up their children's ability to fight off infections (or possibly even cancer).

Finally, when you begin to understand how they work, you may come to this realization: vaccines are just gross. We have fewer McDonald's and more Panera Bread stores everywhere. We have Trader Joe's and Whole Foods everywhere. We have organic food restaurants and Berkee water filters. All because people are more concerned than ever about what is going into their bodies.

If you were to take the ingredients in a vaccine and stick it on the label of a product at Whole Foods, no one would ever buy it. It's not organic. It's unnatural. It is decidedly the opposite of everything that many of us fight for our children every day. The only reason people allow it is because they fear disease more than the vaccine itself. Hopefully, from what I've told you so far, you don't fear the diseases as much as you did.

Chapter 30
Are Vaccines Safe?

With any product, particularly medical products, there can be danger. Within a free and open society, there are two release valves which work in your interest to protect you from harm: safety testing and lawsuits. Reasonable government regulations should require that the product be properly safety tested before being released to the public. Secondly, if a product—despite passing rigorous safety testing—is still causing harm, the company that manufactures that product can be sued for damages—an effect which should both compensate those harmed by the product, and force the manufacturer to fix the problem to avoid future lawsuits. Unfortunately, through purposeful manipulation of the system, neither of these release valves exist as they should with vaccines.

Let's take a quick look at the first issue—safety testing. Vaccines are not classified as drugs and, as a result, can be safety tested much differently than a typical pharmaceutical product. In a drug safety trial, a group of patients are given the true drug and another group are given a placebo—an inert substance that should be incapable of causing a problem, such as saline. The trial might run for months, even years, to discover any negative effects the drug might be causing.

Because vaccines are not considered drugs, their safety trials are run much differently. Rather than looking for problems for months or years, they might look for a few days, and in some cases the trial may only last 48 hours. There is no rule for the minimum amount of time required to look for problems, so they will obviously run the trial for as short of a time as possible. It's infinitely cheaper that way, and problems are much less likely to appear.

If someone in a 48-hour vaccine safety trial began to notice a problem two or three days after they received the vaccine, this event will likely not be considered as caused by the vaccine. The effect of this tiny window of observation is obvious: for a vaccine to be blamed for any safety issue, it has to happen nearly instantaneously—an unlikely occurrence.

A second problem with vaccine safety trials—those conducting the trials claim they can't use a true placebo because it would be unethical. Why? They will say purposefully denying someone a vaccine to protect them from disease is not fair to that person. Despite the fact that the trials run for only days—after which the person would be free to get whatever vaccines they wanted—vaccine manufacturers claim that to deny someone any vaccine for those few days during the trial would be too risky for the patient. So rather than running a useful study by administering half of the group a saline placebo, they administer an existing, already licensed vaccine and compare the results of the new vaccine against that one (a vaccine which was also likely approved under a similarly flawed trial).

This is a practice so asinine you will probably assume that I am attempting to mislead you. You may be thinking, "Maybe this happened once or twice and you're making the suggestion that all trials are run this way." I will ask you to do a study on vaccine trials yourself. Don't trust what I'm saying—look them up yourself and you will find they're nearly all run this way. One large trial testing the much-hated Gardasil vaccine did employ a tiny saline placebo group but relied on an aluminum-only injection for its main placebo.

The inevitable result of these two things is the illusion that every vaccine is safe. The test is unlikely to pick up adverse events due to its short duration, and even if it did, comparing it against another vaccine is likely to create a similar number of problems. If it were compared against a truly inert, saline placebo, the contrast would be much more pronounced.

There are other tricks the clinical trials employ to improve the appearance of safety. They kick out anyone who has any health condition at all. As a result, the health profile of the trial participants doesn't resemble the general population, but a super-human race of perfectly healthy creatures. If someone does develop an issue during the trial, doctors might be encouraged by those running the trial to diagnose the issue in such a way as to appear as if it were a pre-existing condition. If this happens, the participant is kicked out of the trial and their issue is never recorded as a negative event against the vaccine.

One of the most concerning things about these safety trials is they're rarely conducted on babies or pregnant women—the two groups of people most often receiving vaccines and the most vulnerable to their ill effects. You can look through the 25 or so flu vaccines currently licensed in the United States and not a single one of them has ever been safety tested on pregnant women, despite routinely being administered to them. The same holds true for the TDaP shot given to pregnant women. The fact that doctors inject pregnant women with this vaccine every day without a second thought should give anyone nightmares.

Finally, you should know that the vaccine schedule has never been safety tested. Different vaccines have gone through these fraudulent safety trials as standalone products, but never together, as administered. Many babies will receive six, seven, sometimes eight or more vaccines in one visit. Combining so many injections like this without having tested them together would never be attempted with any other pharmaceutical product. The possible interactions between various drugs would be carefully studied and monitored. With vaccines, it's assumed there is no upper limit to the number an infant can receive simultaneously, and the possibility of cross-reactions between their various ingredients has never been studied.

Because of the way vaccine safety trials are conducted now, it wouldn't matter. Even if the full schedule were tested, it would be run as fraudulently as the stand-alone products currently are. It would not be tested against a true placebo, and the trial would run for mere days before being shut down and declared a success.

Again, you are probably having a difficult time believing this is true. I have done the research along with some of the best scientific minds in this field and can assure you, this is the reality of vaccine safety in the United States at this time. Great efforts have been made to raise awareness about the problem, but the pharmaceutical industry is the most powerful lobby in government and is not going to allow proper vaccine safety to be conducted at this time.

I mentioned there were supposed to be two release valves designed to protect consumers from harm regarding potentially dangerous products. The safety trials regarding vaccines are a complete joke and should not be relied on for any meaningful data.

What about the second release valve—lawsuits? If the way in which vaccine safety trials are manipulated doesn't make your blood boil, I can guarantee you the way in which vaccine lawsuits are conducted will.

Chapter 31
Why Vaccine Makers Can't Be Sued

In the 1980s, an increasing number of SIDS (or *Sudden Infant Death Syndrome*) deaths began to be associated with vaccines that had been administered just days—sometimes hours—earlier. While scientists and doctors have never officially declared a cause for babies that die suddenly without any apparent reason, many parents insist that immunizations triggered their baby's death.

The DTP vaccine, long considered to be one of the most dangerous shots, was often implicated. In 1979, four children from Tennessee died within 24 hours of their first DPT shot. It turned out all of the children had received vaccines from the same production batch. Parents were fuming mad and the news media began to pick up on the stories.

Lawsuits began to pile up and vaccine manufacturers saw the writing on the wall—they wouldn't be able to defend themselves from these lawsuits and be able to stay in business. They did something extraordinary that has never happened in any other industry or product—they threatened to cease manufacturing of vaccines if the government couldn't protect them from lawsuits.

Astonishingly, their demands were heard and met. In 1986, a piece of legislation, called the National Childhood Vaccine Injury Act, was signed into law to great fanfare by Ronald Reagan. With the introduction of this new law, vaccine manufacturers could no longer be sued for problems caused by their childhood vaccines—they were protected by the government. It called for the creation of a special court where vaccine injury cases would be heard—again, nothing like this exists in any other industry that I'm aware of.

If the court decides that a death or injury was due to a vaccine, the court will pay out a maximum of $250,000. This money doesn't come from the manufacturers themselves, but a special fee included in the cost of the shot—paid by you each time you or your child receives a vaccine.

Fast-forward 32 years later, and it's clear the court has become a nightmare for parents of children harmed by vaccines. Families are forced to suffer through sometimes years of litigation—all in hopes of getting a maximum of $250,000. Many of these cases never even make it to court because doctors are so insistent the recent appearance of a child's seizures or other problems had nothing to do with vaccines.

The court is very selective in the scientific data it allows and, by all appearances, serves the role of protecting pharmaceutical interests from damage. Although settlements paid by the court are not coming out of the manufacturer's pockets directly, the court's unspoken job is to protect even the appearance of problems with vaccines. If they were to allow many of the plaintiff's cases to win, it would encourage other parents to file their claims. Even so, the court, which hardly anyone is even aware of—even by doctors and nurses—has paid out over $4 billion dollars since it began.

As a result of the 1986 National Childhood Vaccine Injury Act, vaccine manufacturers have been given blanket immunity from any problems their vaccines may cause. Only a fool would believe this would somehow increase the safety of the products they make. In reality, it's done the opposite. Manufacturers have no incentive to properly safety test their vaccines. They can't be sued if something goes wrong, and the safety trials are worse than useless.

Combined with stern recommendations from the government that every child receive vaccines manufacturers can't be sued for, it has created a unique and profitable situation for pharmaceutical companies. No other industry on the planet is afforded this protection—and for good reason. The ability for companies to be punished for creating dangerous products is one of the foundational mechanisms for keeping consumers safe from harm. Imagine the government requiring you to feed your baby a particular formula—breastmilk not allowed—while at the same time preventing you from suing the formula manufacturer for any problems their product caused in your baby. You might really start to wonder who is watching out for you and your child, wouldn't you?

With laughable vaccine safety trials and complete protection from lawsuits, I hope you'll understand why people like me are so reluctant to take vaccine manufacturers and their public health colleagues at their word. After having read about multiple cases of twins dying from SIDS the same night—sometimes the night after their well-child visit, you should really begin to question what might be causing these mysterious deaths. When so many parents have insisted their children came down with other strange problems just days after their vaccines, others are starting to listen. Those who make vaccines, those who administer them, and those who enforce the laws regarding their use may not feel an urge to more thoroughly understand their safety, but I certainly do.

Chapter 32
Will Your Doctor Fire You?

Many mothers ask, "Will my doctor fire me if I skip or delay certain shots?" When they say being *fired*, they mean, will they be asked to leave the doctor's practice. Some doctors will ask you to leave their practice if you deviate from their schedule the tiniest bit. This is horrible, isn't it? You may have a completely valid reason to delay or skip a particular vaccine, but some doctor's offices don't care. You must adhere to the schedule, or else! Before you get upset, don't worry, the next chapter in this book explains how to find a doctor who will work alongside you, rather than against you.

Why would a doctor ask you to leave their practice if you don't adhere to the recommended vaccine schedule exactly? They wouldn't do this for antibiotics—a medicine which could prevent the spread of an *actual* infection rather than a *potential* infection. It's a simple answer, really—there is a lot of money at stake for them—much more than you probably realize. Before I explain, I want to talk about the reason they *say* they're asking you to leave.

They will say that they're concerned for all the other sick children in their practice and they can't take the risk to allow any kids in their offices who aren't properly vaccinated. This is completely false. There are children coming through their office doors every day who may have one of a thousand other bacterial or viral infections that can make us sick, but for which there are *no* vaccines for. What do they do with those children? They ask them to play on the other side of the waiting room. Do they ask them to stay away from the office until they feel better? Do they ask them to put on a mask? No, they ask them to come in and try and stay on the other side of the waiting room.

On the other hand, if your child had their first 2 DTaP shots at 2 months and 4 months, shots that are supposed to work for years by the way, and you decide that maybe two months later at their 6-month-old visit they don't really need a third, well then they'll claim you're putting their patients at risk! You could probably have a medically-supported reason to delay, such as your child was really sick, but even then, they might say, how dare you put our other patients at risk!

What's going on here? Are they seriously that concerned that delaying a third injection of a shot that's supposed to work for years and years is going to cause one of their patients to get sick? No. They're not. It's clear this is a cover for something else. They will say it's to protect their other patients but the reality is it's to protect a very large bonus they receive from their insurance companies.

If a pediatric practice makes sure a certain percentage of their patients are perfectly vaccinated according to the schedule, an insurance company like Blue Cross Blue Shield might pay them $400 per child. At a large practice, that could amount to tens of thousands of dollars at the end of the year. If they drop below the threshold, they lose all the money. *All* of it. So if they're hovering at the threshold and one mom—like say you—comes in and says my kid is really sick and I don't feel comfortable with them receiving vaccines right now (a smart choice by the way), you could cost them tens of thousands of dollars, just because you're making the right decision for your child. The compliance rules don't take into account different edge cases like your child is sick, or they may have had a reaction to a previous shot. They don't care about that—it's too complicated to manage over thousands of patients. These practices must maintain a certain threshold of perfectly vaccinated children or they'll lose their bonus.

Another problem has emerged recently. As mom-and-pop doctor's offices have gotten bought by larger hospitals, their ability to practice medicine independently has disappeared. The larger hospitals have a complex set of compliance rules they have to work within to receive the maximum amount of reimbursements from Medicare and other government programs. These rules trickle down into the pediatric doctor's offices. "Standards of care," they're called. Medical workers are required to enforce these standards of care blindly, and often aren't allowed to use their personal judgement or common sense.

If your pediatric doctor doesn't have the specter of losing their insurance bonuses hanging over their head, they may still have these complex compliance issues they're forced to adhere to because of a larger corporation above them requires it for financial reasons. It's a horrible situation that has caused many doctors to either figure out a way to work independently or leave practicing medicine completely.

Finally, and this may be obvious, but vaccines are many pediatric doctors' most important procedure. Their reputation is largely built upon this one thing—immunizations. It's strange, because it's probably the thing they learn they *least* about in medical school, and it's the thing that takes the *least* amount of knowledge or skill to administer. I think gas station attendants are administering the flu shot nowadays. Anyway, doctors' ability to diagnose hundreds of different diseases or remember which medicines might work for which infections *is* an incredible feat of intelligence, but most would consider the *mystery* of vaccination to be their greatest magic trick. Because of this, you can understand why some of them might be uncomfortable with growing numbers of parents who are skipping vaccines for their children. They may feel threatened that parents might stop bringing their children to them for *anything*. This is obviously not going to happen, but change is hard, especially for those pediatricians that rely so heavily on vaccines.

So don't take it personally if a doctor asks you to leave their practice because you want to delay or skip certain shots. Your decision may cost them tens of thousands of dollars and I'm sure you can understand why they'd be reluctant to keep you around. But don't worry—there are other options. There are more and more physicians making a stand for parental rights every day. Doctors are practicing independently and are again becoming a new mother's health partner rather than their enemy.

Chapter 33
How to Find a Flexible Doctor

If you are thinking of delaying, skipping, or altering the administration of certain vaccines to your child, you will probably need to find a doctor who is willing to work with you. Because increasing numbers of mothers are beginning to push back against so many vaccines for their children, a number of new options are appearing that make having a positive relationship with your pediatrician possible.

One of the first things you might look for in choosing a pediatrician is an independent practice. Because of the bureaucratic burden brought on by the Affordable Care Act, many independent doctors have had to sell their practices to larger, regional hospitals that have the bandwidth to handle all of the new compliance issues. There are still some doctors out there that have managed to remain independent and can more freely act in your best interests. I wouldn't consider it rude to call a pediatrician's office and ask them straight away if they're an independent practice or are owned by another company. As you search for a pediatrician, make that one of your first questions: Are you independent, or owned by someone else? Ask them who specifically. They might be owned by another practice, or a regional hospital. The larger the entity that controls them, the less flexibility they're likely to have in working with you on your decisions.

Next, you will want to go ahead and ask them if they allow adjustments to the vaccine schedule. You may not think you care about this, but believe me, you will. You do not want to get stuck in a relationship where doctors and nurses are pushing a medical procedure onto your baby when your maternal instincts are screaming that something is wrong. If they show any hesitancy at all on this question, I would move on to the next practice. Many doctors and their practices know that mothers are now researching vaccines and want the freedom to make adjustments as they see fit. These practices should answer emphatically, "Yes. We are completely fine with your choices as a parent on vaccination." If you hear confusion, as if they've never been asked, or if they're happy to have your business but don't feel comfortable with where the conversation is headed, walk away. There are always other pediatricians that will work with you rather than against you.

Another new type of pediatric practice that has become popular recently is called *direct primary care*. With these types of practices, you pay a monthly membership fee per child and typically gain unlimited access. People who do this often have catastrophic insurance in case something really bad happens, but for their normal sick kid stuff, they just pay a monthly fee to the practice and are free to go whenever they need to. This is an awesome model that seems to work for both doctors and their patients. Doctors can practice independently without the cloud of insurance compliance hanging over them, while parents save money and usually have much more freedom with the details of their children's care. If you can find a direct primary care pediatrician near you, they would definitely be a good place to start looking for a doctor who's more likely to offer flexibility when it comes to vaccines.

A third option is to take your child to a family care doctor. They're often familiar with the same sorts of milestones and health checks performed at a typical well-child visit but often don't have the insurance compliance issues that a normal pediatrician might. I would still ask them about their independent status and stance on vaccination because this will always factor into your interactions with them.

Another option is to take your child to a pediatric chiropractor. This is not so your infant can have their back adjusted, but because pediatric chiropractors are often trained to recognize behavioral and developmental milestones just like pediatricians. Most pediatric chiropractors don't offer pediatric vaccines as part of their practice. If you're avoiding vaccines altogether and just want the peace of mind of having your baby looked over by a professional for any warning signs you feel you might have missed, consider taking them to a pediatric chiropractor. You'll probably be surprised at the depth of their knowledge and stress-free environment their appointments can provide.

Finally, many parents who have multiple children and have decided to forego most, if not all, vaccines just skip the well-child visits altogether. Because the well-child visits are basically shot visits, most parents with multiple children know what to look for and see no reason to take their infant into an environment that likely has other sick children. If there is something that concerns them, they'll go in for an appointment. If their child is developing fine, there is no reason to see a doctor for a healthy child.

There are many resources online and in books that will provide you with a clear picture of what to expect of your child at different milestones. Whatever you decide, make sure that your pediatrician is willing to work with you, rather than against you. They're capable of exerting enormous pressure to perform medical procedures you may not feel comfortable with. If your child is sick, and you don't want them receiving any vaccines, you don't want to have a fight with your pediatrician over shots when you're concerned about something completely different. Don't budge on this. Spend the extra effort to find a pediatrician that is your ally and your life will be so much easier!

Chapter 34
Should You Sign Vaccine Refusal Forms?

You may have heard stories of parents who declined certain vaccines and were asked by their doctors to sign "Vaccine Refusal" forms. You probably want to know if *you* should sign one of these forms. These documents are completely meaningless, have no legal ramifications (currently) and serve no purpose other than to scare you and to put additional pressure on you to vaccinate *your* children according to the CDC guidelines so that doctors don't miss out on their insurance bonuses for fully vaccinated children. This paper is a way to sniff out "problem" parents so they can dump you and replace your healthy family with a more cooperative mother who won't cost them money.

There is nothing illegal about this document, but there is also nothing illegal about them telling you they don't want your child as a patient if they don't feel like you're going to be perfectly compliant. They could make you sign an "I'll Never Be Late for An Appointment" document or a "I Will Only Give Positive Reviews of this Pediatric Practice on Facebook" document. They can make whatever document they want, ask you to sign it, then refuse you service if you don't. It's a free country, for some, at least. It's a very strange thing obviously, but somehow people have gotten the feeling that for some reason because it's about vaccines, this document has some sort of legal standing. It doesn't. It's just a way to try to pressure and shame you.

Some people feel reluctant to sign it because they might use it against you in the future somehow. I don't really know what that might entail other than providing proof that you are not a fully compliant automaton. You can refuse to sign it, of course, but they may tell you you're not welcome there if you don't. So you can sign it, then continue to have battles with them every time you bring your child in for a well-child visit. If you don't have an alternative at this point, I'd just sign the form, mark out what you disagree with, and initial those places. You could always indicate that you're not refusing vaccines but are going to vaccinate according to "The Healthy Mother" vaccine schedule. *You're* the healthy mother. I'd just tell them it's a popular book if they ask. But that's me. You have to decide what's right for you.

These forms are just a stupid, childish thing for doctor's offices to have even gotten in to. They are the whining of an annoying child that isn't getting his way. If you attend a pediatric office that even has these forms anywhere in their office, I would leave and let them know you don't want your child being seen by physicians who put the needs of their business before the needs of the children they see. As you are searching for a pediatrician's office, this is probably a good way to sniff out practices which are not going to put your family's needs first. Ask them if they make patients sign vaccine refusal forms. If they do, I'd start looking to take your baby somewhere else, right away.

Chapter 35
Vaccines If Your Child is Sick?

Many parents want to know "If my child is sick and they're supposed to get some shots. Should we still go?" If it were my child, there is absolutely no way I would consider a vaccine for them. Vaccines are not supposed to be administered to a child unless they're in perfect—or as close to perfect—health as they can be. Remember that you are purposefully injecting them with modified versions of pathogens that can cause serious problems. You are depending on their immune system to be able to fight these off. Doctors then add another layer by injecting children with multiple vaccines at the same time—as if it's a harmless, risk-free operation. Finally, add to that the stress to a child of being physically restrained by a nurse, or you, their parent, and they might have the beginnings of a serious health event.

If you call the doctor's office on the day of a scheduled well-child visit and let them know your child is sick, then ask them if they should still come in, they will frequently tell you yes. They'll say "if they never vaccinated sick children they'd never vaccinate anyone." This is careless and stupid. For people who won't pay the price if something bad happens to your child, this is easy for them to say. It's kind of remarkable that the folks who work at a doctor's office act terrified for your child to come in if they're one day late getting a particular shot, as if that makes them somehow magically vulnerable to a disease they were just vaccinated for weeks earlier. But if you tell them your child is projectile vomiting, they'll say, "Come on in. We'll get those shots in and they'll be good as new." Strange how it works, isn't it?

Remember, vaccines make your children sick on purpose. Sick with versions of what are considered to be some of the more dangerous infections floating around. So to purposefully subject your children to these injections, particularly multiple ones, while they're *already* sick seems absolutely insane to me.

Being sick while getting vaccines has another concern for me—one that is a bit more complex and I talk about in the autism chapter. When you are sick, your brain signals for help using your immune system. Your brain is the most important part—besides your heart—of your body. So you can understand why when you're sick, your brain signals for help. If you don't already know this, the frontline defense system of your immune system are white blood cells. White blood cells gobble up viruses and bacteria considered to be invaders. They don't just float around randomly throughout your body—they go where they're signaled for help. And when you're sick, your brain sends out all kinds of signals for help. It says to white blood cells "Come here. Help is needed here." Your immune system wants to make sure your brain is protected. Unfortunately, the aluminum that is contained in many shots, gets gobbled up by white blood cells. They think the aluminum is an invader and try to destroy it. But they can't, so they continue to move around, with the aluminum inside them—and remember that aluminum is a neurotoxin. It's very good at destroying neurons in your brain.

I don't know if you see the problem yet, but if you inject aluminum, a neurotoxin, into your body, at *the same time* you are sick, that aluminum is going to get eaten by the white blood cells and the white blood cells are then going to end up getting signaled to your brain. In case it's not clear, you don't want neurotoxins in your brain, and getting vaccinated with aluminum-containing vaccines while sick is the perfect way to do that. If someone tells you that you should bring your child in to get vaccines even though they're sick, I'd tell them to take a hike. There is no infection on this planet scary enough for me to risk that for.

Chapter 36
Should You Spread Shots Out?

If you're like a lot of moms, you might feel like there are too many shots. Because I also feel that way, my goal is to reduce the number of shots necessary as far down as possible. Zero would be ideal. You've probably also seen a scary-looking pictures of trays full of syringes and band-aids. If this image doesn't at least send a little bit of terror through your heart, I don't know what would. It's an awful image. No mother, child, or nurse or doctor for that matter really *wants* to put a child through this. It's a terrible experience—getting so many shots in one visit. Humans have a primal fear of being stabbed with things—it's just a natural response to external things breaking through the surface of our largest organ—our skin.

Because of this, many mom's natural reaction is to spread the shots out so they don't get so many at once. In some ways, this would seem to be good. Our bodies would typically never have to fight off multiple infections at once, and so to space vaccines out in such a way we reduce the number of infections our immune system must battle might seem like a good idea. It probably is a good idea, in one sense, but it introduces another problem—one that I also talk about in the autism chapter.

There are so many shots required of children these days that manufacturers are trying to figure out ways to combine more and more vaccines into one injection. They just approved a new hexavalent vaccine, which combines six of them together. Nurses and parents will love this because it means fewer injections to subject children too, but the tradeoff is 1) children will get more infections to deal with at the same time, and 2) if a problem develops, it will be harder to know specifically what caused the problem.

For me, the real issue with spacing out shots comes from a strange source: fear. I mentioned earlier how being sick and getting vaccines is a horrible idea because when you're sick, your brain starts asking for help from white blood cells. And if you've just been vaccinated with shots that have aluminum, your white blood cells are going to pick up that aluminum and are likely to going to inadvertently deliver some of it directly to your brain. This is *not* good obviously. Another huge trigger that will cause your brain to start signaling for help from white blood cells is fear. The more afraid you are, the more the brain will signal for help. We're not really sure why this is, but it kind of seems obvious that if your body senses danger or that something bad may happen, your brain preemptively begins to signal for help from your immune system—you know, just in case.

When we examine the fear response in humans, you can kind of divide it into two stages. The first is fight or flight. You all have probably heard of that one. Your body tenses up. It raises your heart rate. It starts diverting resources away from digestion and your immune system towards better muscle and brain function. But there is another stage beyond that which kicks in when it appears that fight or flight aren't going to work. This happens when you're immobilized or restrained. When you're immobilized or restrained, and it's obvious you can't fight or flee, your brain *really* starts signaling for help from your white blood cells—white blood cells likely to contain the neurotoxin aluminum. Unfortunately, vaccination, particularly with little toddlers, often creates this very scenario. Sometimes they're sick, of course, but often times—most times—they are afraid. So afraid, they might require immobilization or restraint from mom and a nurse or two. This scenario will cause their brain to signal *hard* for white blood cells to come to their aid—white blood cells likely containing aluminum.

This is a horrible realization to make, but one that explains why toddlers seem to suffer neurological injury from vaccinations more often that babies. Infants have no idea what's coming. They can't recognize danger. Toddlers certainly can. Parents often have to bribe their children with promises of ice cream or toys to make it through a vaccine visit.

Because of this, you can start to see why I feel like spreading out shots might not be as good of an idea as some people think. Once your baby reaches 12 months, and especially around the 15-18 month mark and up, they will be aware of what's happening. They will react with fear, especially if you have to physically immobilize or restrain them. The more often this happens, the more fear they're likely to experience every time. They will have less time to have forgotten about the previous visit and may even start showing anxiety as you pull into the doctor's parking lot.

The complications of having multiple vaccines at once are numerous and something I would avoid if at all possible. If the end result of spacing out shots is that they're delayed until later, when your child is less afraid, then I think that is a good thing, no matter what you decide to. The way in which fear can signal aluminum directly to the brain causes me even more concern. Spreading doctor visits out so that this whole ritual of waiting room, exam room, restraint, then injection, happening over and over again may eventually cause even more problems. For this reason, if you're dead set on administering your child aluminum-containing vaccines, I would *not* do it if it requires restraint or immobilization. Wait until they're older and can understand that you're trying to help them. I would not administer aluminum-containing vaccines in a way that essentially requires violence. Nobody will benefit from that.

Chapter 37
Can Your Children Still Attend Public School?

Many of you are curious about whether your children can still attend public school or daycare if they don't have the full vaccine schedule. In some states, daycare, private or religious schools are thought of separately from public schools and can require whatever they want. In other states, they might have to adhere to whatever the state law requires. Certain church-based organizations may be more relaxed. It's not uncommon to have to do a little searching around to find a facility that is flexible and will accept your super-healthy child into their program. Don't get discouraged—ask around with some local natural health groups. Hang out at the salad bar at Whole Foods and ask some moms there about daycare centers that are "Vaccine Aware."

If you plan to homeschool your child, you are free to do whatever you want, in most states, currently. Some states may require you to fill out an exemption even if you home school, but for now that's probably the easiest route. Home school is not always possible for everyone, obviously, but many families who are not vaccinating end up going that route (for other reasons beside just vaccines). I've heard that California is trying to force even homeschoolers to adhere to the CDC recommended vaccine schedule, but as far as I know, no other states are forcing them to.

There are basically three types of vaccine exemptions you need to know about: personal or philosophical exemptions, religious exemptions, and medical exemptions. All states offer medical exemptions, as these are the most limiting and difficult to obtain. Personal or philosophical exemptions offer the most freedom. With a personal or philosophical exemption, your child can attend public school no matter which vaccines they've had (all, extra, or none) simply because of what you believe. These states offer the most flexibility when it comes to public school and vaccines by offering all three types of exemptions: *Pennsylvania, Ohio, Michigan, Wisconsin, Louisiana, Arkansas, Texas, Oklahoma, Minnesota, North Dakota, Colorado, Utah, Arizona, Idaho, Washington, and Oregon.* If you live in any of these states, you are good to go.

Religious exemptions are offered in many other states. They allow you to object to certain vaccines on religious grounds, such as aborted fetal cell tissue sometimes being an ingredient. As I mentioned, all states offer the restrictive medical exemption, but if you live in any of the following states and can prove your religious affiliation to their standards, you can opt out of any and all vaccines and still have your child attend public school: *Vermont, New Hampshire, Massachusetts, Maine, Rhode Island, Connecticut, New Jersey, Delaware, Maryland, Washington, D.C., Virginia, North Carolina, South Carolina, Georgia, Florida, Indiana, Kentucky, Tennessee, Alabama, Illinois, Iowa, Missouri, South Dakota, Nebraska, Kansas, Montana, Wyoming, New Mexico, Nevada, Alaska, and Hawaii.*

Medical exemptions are the most restrictive, as they rely on doctor's decision to decide whether your child is medically eligible to be exempt from vaccines. Getting a medical exemption can be very difficult, especially in states where this is the only exemption offered. There are four states where medical exemption is the only choice parents have in using a delayed or altered vaccine schedule while still being able to send their children to public school. These are *California, West Virginia, New York,* and *Mississippi*. If you live in one of these four states, you should know that if you plan on sending your children to public school and want to potentially skip certain vaccines, you will have a battle on your hands. The good people in these states are constantly fighting political battles in an attempt to return the other, more flexible exemptions that have been recently taken away from parents. I'd consider trying to help them if you live in one of these states (or live nearby and have extra bandwidth). You will hear horrible stories of children who developed conditions after their vaccines in these states that are still refused medical exemptions despite an obvious injury.

To summarize, if you live in California, Mississippi, New York, or West Virginia and want your children to attend public school, you currently will have to work hard to get a medical exemption. Medical exemptions are hard to obtain in these states. Consider home school, private school, or moving to one of the more flexible states. Political laws do change, so before you do anything drastic, make sure to check the internet to see if your state has changed its law. If you live in the second group of states and have some religious objection to vaccines, you are set. Your child will be able to attend public school without problems. If you live in the first group of states, your public schools will welcome your child no matter what their vaccine status is. Funny that they do this all the time without really any problems and your doctors office might refuse you service for the same thing. That is the situation on public schools and vaccines. Most states have local organizations that can help you with any questions regarding these laws.

The best place to find out the specific laws regarding your state is the National Vaccine Information Center website, which is nvic.org. I'd start there—they will probably have answers to most any of your state specific questions.

Chapter 38
The Meningococcal Vaccine

The meningococcal vaccine is something a lot of parents ask about, so I'm going to go a bit more in depth than I have on some of the others. It's officially recommended at 11-12 years old, and again at 16 years old, so if you're just having a baby, you can probably skip this chapter for now—there's a lot of information to take in. 11-12 years old may not feel like a pediatric vaccine, but pediatric medicine can refer to people as much as 21 years old. We often think of it as young children, but officially, I believe pediatric physicians in the U.S. have determined their care extends to 21. And just so you know about the pronunciation, there are at least two acceptable ways to say it: muh-NIN-juh-cock-uhl OR muh-NIN-GUH-cock-uhl. Juh or Guh. Most people have heard of meningitis, with a J, so I feel more comfortable calling it the muh-NIN-juh-cock-uhl vaccine.

Meningitis, which means a swelling or inflammation of the lining of the brain, is a *symptom*. Many different things can cause it. This causes people a bit of confusion in a similar way that polio does. Polio was originally the name of a symptom. They developed a vaccine for one of the many different microbes that could cause it, and named that particular virus *poliovirus*. Over time, the symptom became associated with that one virus, even though it could be caused by many different ones.

The same thing is happening with the meningococcal vaccine. Meningitis can be caused by many different things—both viruses and bacteria—even funguses, occasionally. They've developed a vaccine that targets one of the microbes that can cause it, and so they had to name the infection caused by that particular bacteria. They call it *meningococcal* disease. Just to confuse things, you'll occasionally hear the term *bacterial* meningitis. This can mean meningitis caused by one of several different types of bacteria—not only the vaccine one, but any bacterial infection that caused meningitis. Bacterial meningitis is usually more several than viral meningitis, which can be caused by several different viruses.

Got it? Meningitis is a symptom. There is *viral* meningitis—caused by one of many viruses. Fungal meningitis caused by a fungi. And bacterial meningitis—swelling of the lining of the brain caused by the infection of one of many different types of bacteria. Meningococcal *disease* is meningitis caused by that one bacteria they've developed a vaccine for. So there are probably a hundred things than can cause meningitis, and at least four bacteria that can cause it: pneumococcus, haemophilus, listeria, and meningococcus. The vaccine we're talking about protects against one of those bacteria—the meningococcus bacteria. And to confuse things further, there are several different strains of this particular meningococcus bacteria which vaccines might target.

The pneumococcus bacteria can create a particularly nasty bacterial infection, which is why they developed a vaccine for it. The infection can cause swelling of the brain but gets really bad when it gets into the bloodstream. This bacteria creates a poison called an *endotoxin*, which is a poison that exists inside the bacteria.

These poisons don't really affect you until the bacteria and the toxin is released from inside the cell. If you have an aggressive meningococcus infection and take antibiotics, this might cause a massive cell die-off, which can cause a massive release of those endotoxins. This is what causes sepsis, swelling, and those really awful looking blue and black limbs you may have seen scary pictures of.

When most people get a meningococcus infection, they don't even realize it. Many children have already developed immunity to it by the time they hit twelve or thirteen years old. For reasons we don't understand, some people react poorly to it. If you smoke, or live with someone who smokes, your baby is much more likely to have a problem with this infection. If you live in crowded, unsanitary conditions or your baby has another illness, they're also much more likely to have a problem clearing this infection.

There are six different kinds of meningococcal disease vaccines licensed in the United States. Three of them cover 4 of the more common strains of the meningococcus bacteria (A, C, Y, and W), two of them cover a type B strain—which seems to be more common amongst younger children—and the last one covers C and Y but is combined with a HIB vaccine. I'd forget about the B and combined shots and just remember the 4-strain A-C-Y-W one—that's the one you'll need to think about. None of the meningococcal vaccines are recommended for anyone under 10 unless there are extenuating circumstances like a rare blood disorder, a problem with their spleen, HIV, etc.

Meningococcal disease can be horrible, so the question is, should your child get this shot? Most women have picked up these different strains without knowing it and can pass on maternal antibodies to their children to help protect them when they're younger, and as a result, the vaccine isn't suggested for infants. At 11-12 years old, doctors will recommend your child receive one of those 4-strain A-C-Y-W meningococcal vaccines, then again at 16 years old. The reason they need another, is because like many other shots, it just doesn't seem to work that well. In fact, it works just over 50% of the time, and even then, just for a few years. If you are really concerned, you could get a titer test for those 4 strains of the bacteria to see if your child has already developed immunity to them without you knowing—chances are good they have.

Children that develop really aggressive cases of this type of bacterial meningitis usually have an underlying condition that predispose them to it. Thankfully, it's extremely rare for a healthy adolescent teen to develop serious problems from a meningococcus infection. Normally, with a vaccine that works this poorly, they would add aluminum as an adjuvant to help give it a boost, but for some reason, the three 4-strain meningococcal shots don't contain aluminum. However, because the likelihood my child hasn't already developed immunity to the A-C-Y or W strains of this particular bacteria is low, and the likelihood they get the aggressive form of this infection is so infinitesimally small, I would skip this shot with no hesitation. If they had some underlying medical condition or if I smoked or we lived in horrible conditions and I was really concerned about it, I would go to one of these AnyLabTestNow type places and get my child's titers checked to see if they had already developed immunity to these different meningococcus strains. If from the test results, it appeared they hadn't developed immunity to those strains, I might consider giving them this shot. Because it works so poorly, I would probably still skip it and would focus on boosting their immune system through good nutrition, a stress-free school experience, and all the other usual suspects.

Chapter 39
The HPV Vaccine

If you have a daughter, she will likely be recommended a vaccine for HPV when she turns 11 or 12. HPV stands for *human papillomavirus*. There are around 200 strains of HPV at last count. It's a common virus that is spread almost exclusively through sexual contact. It can occasionally be passed from mother to child as well as from surgical instruments.

The reason a vaccine was developed for HPV is because some of these strains are associated with cervical cancer. There are other types of cancer that occasionally show up, as well as what are called genital warts, but the real target is cervical cancer. If you get an infection from any of the 200 strains of HPV, you won't even know you have it—it doesn't create a fever or rash, and the infections resolve themselves in 90-95% of people. The most common symptom, warts, come from two HPV strains.

The easiest way to know if you've had an HPV infection is by getting a Pap smear. Pap smears test for 2 of the HPV strains most commonly associated with this type of cancer. According to the American Cancer Society, cervical is the most preventable AND treatable cancer there is. Routine Pap smears will indicate you may have an infection. If you've developed lesions on your cervix, these are easily and routinely removed by a variety of surgical methods. If you get regular PAP smears, you would have to be *extremely* unlucky to get cervical cancer. You'd have to have multiple tests that missed an infection, year after year, or never get a pap smear at all, probably the leading cause of death due to cervical cancer.

There are two vaccines available for HPV—Cervarix and Gardasil. You may have heard of Gardasil both because they run a lot of commercials for it—and because it has a fairly bad reputation for causing problems. These are two relatively new vaccines that have come on the market in the last decade or so. Because cervical cancer often takes some 30 years to develop from an HPV infection, they haven't actually been able to test if the HPV vaccines work. They've tested them against what are called *surrogate endpoints*—things that indicate cancer *might* one day develop. It will likely be another 10 to 15 years before we can definitively say whether the HPV vaccine actually works or not.

For protection from something that is transmitted sexually, it might seem like they're recommending the HPV vaccines a little early. The reason they do this is once you get the HPV infection naturally, the vaccine won't work—you have to catch it before then. But there's another problem that's recently emerged—if you get an HPV vaccine *after* you've already been exposed, it has the unpleasant ability to *increase* the likelihood you will develop cancer —by 44%. Disease enhancement, it's called, and this isn't tinfoil hat conspiracy stuff—the FDA has admitted this phenomenon happens. For some reason, although HPV is very common, they've started recommending it for adults—despite that 44% increased risk of it progressing into cancer (and a 3 times higher rate of miscarriage).

Should your daughter get this vaccine? Well, for starters, we're not sure it works at all, and if she's already got one of these strains of HPV somehow, it might increase her odds of getting cancer. But that's not the real problem—the real problem is there is something very strange going on with these two HPV vaccines that we don't understand. Cervarix and Gardasil are called *recombinant DNA vaccines*, and they're very different than other shots. While they both may contain a type of aluminum, they use them in a heavily modified form that is unlike anything else out there.

The HPV virus is a strange microbe. It's very weak and difficult to replicate in the lab. Because of this, they've had to genetically modify the virus in order to make the vaccine. Apparently, the normal aluminum adjuvant many other vaccines use doesn't work in these types of vaccines, so they've had to create an esoteric version of the adjuvant. It still uses various forms of aluminum but combines them with other things to get enough of a boosting effect. There have been reports of premature ovarian failure, seizures, even death after receiving these HPV vaccines, but thankfully those are rare. Fainting, chronic pain, and other neurological issues seem to be fairly common and are most definitely *not* rare. In fact, more HPV related problems are logged in the VAERS database than all other pediatric vaccines combined. Does it have something to do with the recombinant DNA vaccine itself? Possibly. There was one other of this type of esoteric vaccine—a Hepatitis B vaccine—but it has been pulled from the market and replaced with another manufacturer's more common version. Hepatitis B vaccine-related deaths have gone down since then. Coincidence? You decide.

Is this safe? Unfortunately, we don't know. The vaccine—as it's administered to girls today—has never been safety tested. When they ran the safety trials, it appears the manufacturers manipulated the ingredients to make the vaccines—and placebos—less likely to cause problems. In one small trial in young teens, the vaccine contained *half* the amount of the adjuvant girls receive today. Why?

No one knows. In one Danish safety trial, girls were told it was *not* going to be a safety trial and that some of them would receive an inert placebo. Neither of these things were true—it was a safety trial, and the placebo they received was not inert.

For anyone who has studied the Gardasil safety trials, it feels obvious they're trying to hide something. There are too many strange manipulations, obfuscations, and what feel to be downright lies for me to believe they don't know that something bad is going on with these vaccines. Fertility has gone down by half in some countries where this vaccine is frequently administered. Coincidence? I don't think so. Would I let my daughter have this shot? No way. Absolutely no way. As a parent, I'd be more terrified of this vaccine than the infant hepatitis B shot, which I'm definitely terrified of. If I had a daughter and there was a law that said there was only one pediatric vaccine I could skip, the HPV would be it—by a mile.

You'll notice that they're trying to get boys to get this vaccine now, presumably to protect them from some completely obscure cancers that are most commonly associated with what is called risky sexual behavior. Fill in the gap as to what that means if you don't already know. And just so you know, the vaccine is *not* approved for penile, throat, head and neck cancers. Regardless, they're pushing the HPV vaccine for not only girls, but boys and adults. To me, this feels like a hail Mary, a last ditch attempt to wring a bit more money out of a vaccine that will probably—in my opinion—be off the shelves within a decade. If I had a daughter or son, this would be the number one vaccine I would skip, over all of the others.

Chapter 40
What If Your Doctor Tells You Differently

"But my doctor said vaccines were safe!"

"My doctor said all of her children got their vaccines and nothing happened to them!"

This is probably the most common refrain of anyone who has just begun to question vaccines. Doctors—the ultimate authority on vaccines, right? Who could know more about vaccines than doctors, the ones who administer them every day? I did some research into this and was shocked at what I discovered.

The fact that nothing happened to their children is not surprising. Problems from vaccines don't happen to everyone, and even when something does happen, it might be weeks, even months later. Either way, vaccines are almost never blamed, even when there's an obvious connection. I have seen parents proudly declare their children as the recipients of having safely undergone vaccination with no problems, despite their obvious eczema and ongoing gut issues—two known side effects of vaccines.

Doctors say vaccines are safe because they're taught they're safe. Until something happens to a doctor's own children—when they see their child change overnight after a vaccine—they will insist that vaccines are nearly incapable of causing harm. The horrible irony is that many of the illnesses they attempt to treat every day can be traced back to reactions to a vaccine, a topic I cover in-depth in another book of mine called Crooked:Man-made Disease Explained—a book about how the crooked smiles and misaligned eyes people often see their children develop after vaccines are just the tip of the iceberg of vaccine damage.

If your child starts on an antibiotic and later that day develops hives or nausea, you can guarantee the doctor is likely to take your child off that antibiotic and try something else. If your child receives multiple vaccines and begins having seizures that next day, your doctor is likely to tell you it has nothing to do with the shots and is just a coincidence. If you press them hard and ask them to figure out why your child is suddenly having seizures, they're likely to tell you, "Sometimes we just don't know why these things happen."

Doctors are reluctant to admit vaccines cause problems because a couple of reasons: For one, they have no other tools at their disposal to try and prevent disease. If your child has problems with a particular antibiotic, there are almost always many others they can try—it's the same for most other medicines. However, if your child appears to react poorly to a vaccine, the doctor is out of options for protective care.

Another reason they don't like pointing at vaccines as the source of a problem—their side effects can last forever. When you stop taking medicines, both the effects and side effects generally stop. Because a vaccine's effects are supposed to last for many, many years, the side effects also can. If something bad happens to your child after vaccines, doctors have very few options to deal with it. Doctors know this and are obviously going to point towards something other than what *they* did as the cause for that traumatic event. It's human nature—I might do the same thing.

Finally, the really strange thing about doctors (and nurses) and vaccines—they aren't taught much about them in school. Hardly anything, actually. Compared to the hundreds of hours someone like me has spent studying vaccines, most health care providers know next to nothing. They learn a lot about disease and the immune system and assume that vaccines interact similarly. Unfortunately, they don't. As I mentioned about the ACT problem with the whooping cough vaccine, they're very different. Physicians may spend a few hours learning the schedules recommended by the government, and spend a few hours learning which vaccines should be administered subcutaneously (under the skin) as opposed to intra-muscularly. Beyond that, they learn almost nothing about vaccines.

I was so confused by hearing this, I bought every book listed on the medical curriculum of a prestigious medical school. I even bought some auxiliary books that were not required but on the optional, "recommended" reading list. After going through each and every book on the list—over thousands and thousands of pages—there were only 4 pages that talked about how vaccines work! There were 11 pages that listed the vaccine schedule recommended by the government, but besides that, 4 pages that talked about vaccines.

I made a video about it—showing the books and how little a prestigious medical school's curriculum spent teaching about vaccines. Many doctors and nurses got in touch with me to confirm this had been their experience in medical school. Of course students learn more than what is taught from their schoolbooks, but I imagine the disparity continues into their classroom and residencies.

Once I understood that doctors and nurses learn very little about vaccines in school, I began to realize why they're so hostile to people like myself who ask honest questions about them. I've written books on the subject, but there are many, many amateur vaccine-aware mothers and fathers out there who are much smarter than me. Any of us could easily stump an average pediatric doctor or nurse on vaccines with our knowledge of vaccines.

This isn't to brag in any way on our intellect, because doctors are some of the smartest people I know—it's simply to indicate how little they actually know about vaccines in particular. If we were to have a contest on anatomy, disease, or which drug to use for a certain problem, physicians would absolutely have me beat. When it comes to vaccines, unfortunately even a moderately informed parent is likely to know much more than they do.

I understand that this is going to be very hard for you to accept. Doctors are held high up on a pedestal and we place so much faith in them as they take care of our children. It's a sad state of affairs that the thing they inject into nearly every child that comes into their office, many, many times, whether they're sick or not—they know almost nothing about. This ignorance is usually visible when you question them about the particulars of a vaccine as anger or frustration.

They may tell you the horror story of a child that had tetanus or pneumonia—something they may have seen years ago in their residency at an ER—as anecdotal evidence of the horrors of vaccine preventable disease. This is a blatant attempt to scare you into vaccinating, and it often works. Many parents are unprepared for the amount of bullying they're likely to encounter when even trying to delay a single vaccine. It's a horrible relationship doctors have established with their pediatric parents when honest questions about vaccines are so routinely attacked and met with anger. If your doctor or nurse responds in this way, clearly, they don't have your child's best interests in mind. I would snatch your child from the room and not look back. Your doctor is working for you and your child, not the other way around. They won't have to deal with the ill effects of a vaccine gone wrong. In fact, they would profit from it.

To summarize, doctors and nurses know very little about vaccines. They are taught they're safe and effective and side effects are a one in a million occurrence. If you spend even a short amount of time studying them, you will have already gained more knowledge about vaccines than most medical school students will have.

Chapter 41
What About Herd Immunity?

Herd immunity. It's a term that's thrown around like a weaponized guilt trip. They'll tell you, "Okay, you may have unvaccinated kids, but the only reason you're able to safely do that is because everyone else is vaccinating theirs."

Herd immunity is not what you've been told. I'm going to explain why, but just think about this for a minute: tetanus is not a contagious disease. You can't "spread" it, and you can never develop immunity to it. But the vaccine is required for many jobs, schools, or summer camps—supposedly because of herd immunity!

We've already seen how the threat of most infections had plummeted to nearly zero before many vaccines were invented. The paralysis of polio was related to massive pesticide poisoning and isn't a problem in countries that use safer pesticides. There are very few infections that pose a danger in a first-world country with modern healthcare. People like me strive for as few vaccines as possible—not because they rely on others getting vaccines, but because they don't fear common childhood infections. They know how to treat them if their children do happen to get one, and they're thoroughly informed about the risks of side effects from shots.

Another common herd immunity statement: "You must get your child vaccinated to protect the weak and vulnerable from disease." This is a very powerful argument that attempts to appeal to your civic duty and the natural human compassion we all have. In reality, it doesn't play out the way most people think.

For starters, there are very few people who are truly "immune compromised," meaning their immune systems are so weakened that they cannot receive vaccines. When I say very few, I mean almost none. Statistically speaking, you'd be lucky to encounter more than one in the course of a year of your life. If you were to encounter one of them, you would also have to simultaneously be infected—and not just infected, but infected at the stage where you are capable of transmitting the disease to other people (which is usually just a small window of time within the course of infection). If all of these things lined up, you might inadvertently get someone sick.

Unlikely to ever happen, but again, this call to protect the weak and vulnerable is constantly announced as a reason your healthy child should receive dozens of vaccines—not just to protect them, but the immune compromised around them.

There's a big problem with this—some vaccines can inadvertently trigger the very disease they're designed to protect against. This is because some vaccines contain a modified version of the live virus. If you get vaccinated for a disease with a live virus, you are purposefully creating an infection. Ideally, it's a very mild form of the disease, but sometimes, things go wrong and the vaccine will cause a full-blown infection and become contagious—a phenomenon called *shedding*. This is not a completely obscure event, and in fact, is the main source of polio in many countries today—from the vaccine itself!

You may already be aware of this concept but don't realize it. If you go to any children's cancer ward, you're likely to see a giant warning sign at the entrance warning anyone who has recently been vaccinated to stay away. They know that some vaccines can shed and create the very infection they were intended to protect against. So much for vaccines protecting the weak and vulnerable!

The final plea you hear about herd immunity involves the number of people that have to be vaccinated to keep deadly outbreaks of a disease from happening. For measles, they constantly say at least 95% of country needs to be vaccinated to keep this "horrible" disease at bay.

A few years ago, there was a measles outbreak that started in California's Disneyland. It was blamed on anti-vaxxers causing the number to drop below 95%. No one died, and of the 150 or so people that became infected, over half of them were fully vaccinated for measles—a curious fact that wasn't mentioned in the news.

I want to explain why the herd immunity concept is completely ignored by people like me. Herd immunity originally started as a concept to try to talk people into getting the measles vaccine. In the 1960s, they had just finished developing the measles shot, and because it was considered such a trivial disease that no one was afraid of, no one wanted the vaccine. Scientists did some math and calculated that if just 55% of people were to get the measles vaccine, they could eradicate the disease within two years. Vaccinate 55% of people, and the remaining 45% wouldn't even matter—the disease could be eradicated.

Remember, measles was a minor disease—no one feared it. There were very few deaths because of it, but it was a nuisance—missing school, etc. So they thought eradication would be possible if they could hit the herd immunity number. After a few years of hard work, they were able to hit their vaccination target of 55%. But measles *didn't* go away like they thought it would. People were still getting infected. So they upped the number to around 70%. Eventually, they were able to hit 70% of people vaccinated, and *that* didn't seem to do the trick either. Since then, health authorities have continued raising the herd immunity number to 80%, then 85%, then 90%, then to 95%—where we're at today. Between 90 and 95% of the U.S. has been vaccinated for measles for a long time, yet we still see measles outbreaks. What's going on? Why isn't herd immunity working like we thought?

The main reason is vaccines don't work as long as they had hoped. Natural immunity seems to protect for your entire life—at least long enough that it's really difficult to even test. For vaccines, current estimates range anywhere from 5 to 10 years. It's different for everyone. A natural measles infection used to mean you would never transmit the disease. Now, because only children are getting vaccinated for measles—and the vaccine doesn't protect for more than 10 years—that leaves a significant part of population vulnerable to measles. If only kids get vaccinated, that means everyone else over fifteen years old (and who didn't catch measles as a child) is likely susceptible to measles. That's 80 or 90% of the population that is actually unprotected from measles—right now.

One of the other big problems with vaccines and herd immunity is the way in which certain vaccines mask symptoms of the disease. If you get whooping cough, the build-up of fluid in your lungs will cause you to hack violently in an attempt to get it out. This is a very handy way of mother nature letting you know you are sick. The whooping cough vaccine may prevent you from coughing as much, but it doesn't do much to prevent you from spreading the bacteria. You're still just as infected—and capable of infecting other people—whether you had the vaccine or not.

If you didn't get the vaccine and caught whooping cough, mother nature will give you an obvious warning—violent coughing—a sign that you need to stay away from other people. If you had the vaccine recently, you may be infected, but would have no idea you were carrying a dangerous bacteria. This is why I believe having friends and family members vaccinated for whooping cough before handling babies is very dangerous. I *want* you to know that you're sick. I *want* you to be able to listen to mother nature's warning cues that you shouldn't be handling a baby.

Every vaccine is different, but there are others that cause similar problems and mask the symptoms of the disease so that you might not realize you're infected. The 95% herd immunity threshold is a meaningless number that's been raised many times with no change in measles outbreaks. China raised the number to 100% in their country for many years and continued to see cases of measles. And remember, that number was originally claimed as capable of eradicating the disease. Now they say we need it just to control outbreaks. If the vaccine protected indefinitely, or every single person got a vaccine every 5 years, it might start to make a difference. For a trivial disease like measles, a once in a lifetime natural infection (with essentially zero risk) sounds like a much better option to me.

In summary, when it comes to herd immunity, it hasn't ended up working the way doctors thought it would. Many vaccines don't work for long enough to make a true difference, and many vaccines don't protect against the spread of disease, anyway. If all vaccines could prevent the spread of disease, and they worked for more than a few years, perhaps herd immunity might actually work.

As it stands, every vaccine and every disease are different. Some don't work at all, others work in a very limited way, and still others actually work against the herd immunity concept. This is a lot to take in, but it's important that you understand the truth about herd immunity. It's used as an excuse for so many unnecessary vaccines by people who mean well but are horribly misinformed.

Chapter 42
Should You Give Your Children Tylenol Before/After Shots?

If your child gets a vaccine, they're probably not going to feel very good. Infants are likely to be extra fussy and irritable. Children may run fevers and not want to go to school. Nurses will tell you to give them some Tylenol to help them lower their fevers so they feel better. Online, I've seen mothers PRE-medicating their children hours before their shots with Tylenol in hopes of heading off these problems beforehand.

If this were my child, I would never, ever do this. I think it is incredibly dangerous unless your baby's fever is running high enough to cause them to have seizures. Think about it, vaccines are purposefully giving your child an infection. The job of vaccines is to create a response so that your child's immune system is ready for a *real* infection in the future. When you get sick, part of that immune response is your body raises its internal temperature to help kill of the virus or bacteria. Recent research suggests these fevers aren't "cooking" microbes dead, as was often assumed, but are creating internal changes in your immune system that make it more effective. Regardless, this is all part of a natural system of events your body is designed to execute in order to heal and develop immunity.

Having a fever feels awful—it makes babies super cranky and irritable. But it's a necessary response to infection. It's specifically the major component in how your body is supposed to fight off infection. When you give your sick child Tylenol, it's reducing the fever so that they feel better. The problem is, they cannot fight off the infection (or multiple infections) you injected them with properly. The vaccine is a cheat, a hack to try and give them immunity without the uncomfortable effects of a natural infection. When you add Tylenol to the mix and attempt to suppress the infection—the very thing their body is trying to do to fight off the infection or *infections* they were just given, you may be just increasing the odds of something else going very wrong.

You may have heard that heavy use of Tylenol during pregnancy has been shown to be associated with autism. You may have *also* heard that heavy use of Tylenol during an infant's life has been shown to be associated with autism. These are recent studies that are giving us some indication as to their relationship, even though we don't clearly understand it yet. There are studies associating Tylenol with asthma and rhinoconjunctivitis and eczema. We don't know exactly how these things work together, but apparently there is some sort of tie.

If you're going to give your baby a bunch of vaccines at once, then pump them with Tylenol so they don't feel so bad afterwards, you are really minimizing the chance they can respond properly to the infection. Nothing in life is free. Everything has a cost. You can not—even with vaccines—generate immunity to an infection without some cost. Vaccines sometimes have side effects, and even if they don't they will make your children feel very sick sometimes. To try and squash that sick feeling with Tylenol (or any other fever-reducer) is a very bad idea in my mind. Obviously, I can't speak to you and your child's specific situation, but for me, I would never give my sick child Tylenol unless their fever was so high they were having seizures.

Chapter 43
What About Autism & Vaccines

Do vaccines cause autism? That is the question on many parents minds these days. If you have a new child, especially if it's a boy, and are going to vaccinate them, that is the big cloud that's probably hanging over you. I've studied this subject exhaustively, and am fairly certain I know why vaccines are so frequently associated with autism. I've got a whole book on this if you're interested in reading more about it, but I'm going to summarize what I believe for you here.

Autism is basically defined as two things: impaired social behavior and repetitive patterns of thought or behavior. In reality, there are many other things that are often associated with autism, such as intestinal problems or being sensitive to certain noises. Although there were certainly cases here and there in medical literature of people experiencing these symptoms in the last two hundred years, they didn't appear as isolated symptoms, and in large groups of children, until the 1930s. A physician and psychiatrist, thought of as one of the world's leading experts on childhood psychiatric disorders, started seeing these kinds of children the 1930s. He had never seen them before, and they were all remarkably alike. He'd just written a 500-page paper on all the different childhood mental illnesses he'd seen but there was nothing in his entire book that resembled autism. For him, and the rest of the world, it was something new.

If you haven't been following the genetic search for autism, it's basically a dead end. They've poured hundreds of millions of dollars into looking for a genetic marker for autism and thirty or forty years later, they've found a single marker that is present in about 5% of cases. Since that time, they have discovered the genetic origins many other obscure mental illnesses. Obscure ones you've never heard of with tiny amounts of money for research compared to autism. They found the genetic origin because they were there. Autism apparently does not have a genetic origin, or at least one significant enough for us to find, despite decades and hundreds of millions of dollars in research looking, so that leaves us with an environmental source. An environmental source means that it must be something in our food, the air, or possibly, our medicine.

You may have heard there was a recent scientific study that looked at the amount of aluminum in the brains of several people diagnosed with autism. Their brains contained more aluminum than any others the scientists had ever measured—more than even Alzheimer's patients, who were the previous record-holders. Many people had already started to become concerned about the autoimmune connection with aluminum, but now there are neurological concerns as well.

What most people don't know is that the first time aluminum was added to a childhood vaccine was in 1932. Up until that point, aluminum had never been injected into children. And autism had never been reported. Within a year of children getting that aluminum-containing vaccine, the first cases of what we now call autism began to appear. For those of us who study vaccines, we joke that according to those who administer them, vaccines are the leading cause of coincidence. Autism appearing out of nowhere a year within children getting the first aluminum-containing vaccines is a coincidence too large for me to ignore.

Without going into the details, I'm fairly certain the aluminum many vaccines contain is capable of damaging the brainstem enough to cause autism. Scientists have looked at the relationship between the MMR vaccine (which doesn't contain aluminum) and thimerosal, the mercury the shot *used* to contain and said there was no relation. This is what people are talking about when they say hundreds of studies have proven there is no link between autism and vaccines. If you ask for their sources, most of them look at a single vaccine, the MMR vaccine, and an ingredient it used to contain—mercury. I don't think there are hundreds. There are a good number of studies, but as far as I know, they haven't looked at other vaccines, and they've never looked at aluminum.

I believe a curious phenomenon can happen with the MMR vaccine. Many parents have reported their child regressing into autism after the MMR shot, which *doesn't* contain aluminum. How could that be? There are two very different things that might be happening. With the aluminum-containing vaccines, I believe the neurotoxin can wind up in the brainstem and damage some of the neural pathways that control sensory response and stimulation. Sometimes they're damaged beyond repair and you end up with muted sensory responses. Other times, as these lesions try to heal, they heal incorrectly and can cause over-stimulation. It's difficult to talk about without going into a two-hour explanation, but just understand that the aluminum is perfectly capable of causing the kinds of brainstem injuries that can cause autism.

From my research, I believe that any traumatic event, like getting pinned down to a table and injected with vaccines, can trigger the fear response in the brainstem so aggressively that it signals for help from white blood cells in your body. If the child has received other aluminum-containing vaccines, the metals from those previous shots may get carried into their brainstem, causing the damage that manifests itself as autism.

The MMR shot is frequently administered around the one-year or later mark, when children begin to really become afraid of the doctor's office and restraint or immobilization becomes necessary. If the child already has metals in their body, the timing of this particular shot may be as much of a factor as anything else. But there is something peculiar about the MMR shot that I think is different than any other shot—a difference why I believe it may be so frequently associated with autism. The measles has a tendency to cause encephalitis in the brain. The measles virus in the MMR vaccine is a live virus, and usually doesn't cause many problems. Sometimes the virus isn't properly killed and creates the encephalitis of a typical measles infection. With a natural infection, this would be extremely rare, but because the virus is injected into a screaming, restrained toddler, the nature of the immune system draws that virus into the brain.

Let me explain why this happens. The white blood cells in your body are the soldiers of your immune system. They attack invaders. They also take orders from your immune system, and go where they're signaled to go. They don't just float around randomly looking for trouble, but can go where your body asks for help. If you get an infection from a bacteria or virus, your brainstem signals for help from these white blood cells. If you get a cut or injury, your brainstem signals for help from these white blood cells. And if you are extremely afraid, your brainstem signals for help from these white blood cells. All of these three things happen during vaccination.

Normally white blood cells going to your brain wouldn't be a problem—it would be a good thing. When white blood cells contain aluminum, which is what happens after you get injected with the metal, you don't want them going to your brain, but with the act of vaccination—injury from the injection, infection from the vaccine itself, and the fear of being injected—all three triggers are created. With an MMR injection, even though it doesn't contain aluminum, it does create all three triggers and is likely to transport the measles virus directly into your brain.

If this happens, and the virus has not been properly killed, your child might develop encephalitis, or brain swelling. When this happens to an infant, they'll probably just scream in pain—they're too young to lose the ability to talk or communicate. But when it happens to someone a year old, you might see symptoms that appear just like autism. In fact, something like this happens to adults sometimes. It's called *autoimmune encephalitis*, and it can create some really strange psychological behaviors. I had a friend it happened to, a grown adult, and he changed overnight into someone very different than I had ever known. It was really horrible. Thankfully, he recovered and is back to normal. In children, if this infection persists for weeks or even months, I believe it can cause permanent damage with neurological development.

Even though the mechanism of injury is slightly different, it's safe to call both of them autism. Since the 1970s, women in England were prescribed an epilepsy drug called sodium valproate and would frequently give birth to children with autism. It wasn't a vaccine, and it may not have been the exact same problem, but it *was* autism, just like brainstem damage from aluminum or the encephalitis of the MMR.

Vaccines don't always cause autism, of course, and autism isn't always caused by vaccines. At this point, it's safe to say that vaccines can cause autism. We can debate how often it happens, but to say that vaccines *never* or *have never* caused autism is silly. There are people who may *say* that, but the number of people who actually *believe* that has to be close to zero.

There's a reason populations of children that are mostly unvaccinated, like the Amish, or homeschool children, have such a low rate of autism. It's not because homeschool children are genetically different than others. It's not because the Amish don't take sodium valproate for their epilepsy. It's because both groups tend to get less vaccines than others, and their lowered autism rates show it.

Chapter 44
Are Vaccines and Allergies Related?

Did you know that before vaccines were invented, we didn't even have the word allergy? Before we started injecting foreign material into our bodies, there wasn't a word for anaphylaxis?

Isn't that interesting? How did these words enter into our vocabulary? Allergy is described as "a condition in which the immune system reacts abnormally to a foreign substance." Anaphylaxis describes a very severe allergic reaction to something. It can be life threatening.

There are very few medical conditions that threaten to kill your child multiple times *every* day of their life like a sever food allergy can. Want to send your child to a birthday party? Could be life threatening. Going to a family Thanksgiving meal out of town? Could be life threatening. Every day, every few hours—parents of children with severe food allergies face these decisions. It's exhausting to know a single slip up could end up with the death of your child. Food allergies, and specifically the peanut allergy, are a horrible thing. No child, no parent should have to deal with this problem. There isn't a military prison on earth that could create this kind of long-term psychological trauma.

Before doctors invented words for allergy or anaphylaxis, the only thing similar thing they could talk about was insect stings.

They could sometimes cause a very severe reaction—much more severe than seemed normal. And not coincidentally, insect bites and stings involved an injection of a foreign material into your bloodstream, where your body would create antibodies to it. The next time your immune system encountered that invader—Boom! A massive reaction to attack it—severe enough to kill you. Thankfully, our immune system is designed so well that it requires a very rare situation to cause this type of response. Our gut is very good at keeping most everything out of our bloodstream that shouldn't be there, an incredible feature of our body.

Humans had come along through thousands of years of documented history with apparently nothing resembling allergy. When did it first pop up? The smallpox vaccine. Some children would respond extremely violently to the vaccine. Rashes, like eczema could appear locally, sometimes all over their body, sometimes resulting in death. This was probably one of the nastiest side effects of the smallpox vaccine, and one of the large reasons it was discontinued in the 1970s—*not* because small pox was eradicated, by the way.

No one really knew why this was happening but another shot came along and scientists began to figure it out. It was the diphtheria antitoxin- what's now the "D" in the DTaP and TDaP shots. They would inject a horse with increasing doses of the diphtheria bacteria until it had developed a lot of antibodies in its blood. They would bleed the horse, filter out the red blood cells and take the remaining liquid, optimistically referred to as "serum" and inject it into children in hopes of protecting them from diphtheria. There is a problem here, if you can't see it already. The horse blood contained a million other things in it—things which were never supposed to end up in the blood of children.

The first response to having this diphtheria antitoxin, or horse blood serum, injected into a child's body could sometimes create a mild response but the second one would often create a massive, life threatening reaction. Doctors were very concerned. They didn't know it at the time, but the first injection had resulted in minor side effects as the immune system created antibodies to the foreign material. But the second injection created a violent response that was terrifying. During the research of this phenomenon, French and German scientists coined two new terms to describe what was going on—allergy and anaphylaxis. Doctors even coined a slang term for it: *Serum sickness*, for the liquid they'd harvested from horse blood. And it wasn't 1 in a million. For the diphtheria antitoxin, it was over 40%, according to public health officials at the time.

If you ever wonder if there were always food allergies everywhere, you don't have to wonder. They used to not exist—any allergy, actually as far as I can tell, besides insect bites. And the way we discovered them was through vaccination.

Chapter 45
What Kind of Side Effects Do Vaccines Cause?

You've probably noticed by now that I haven't mentioned much about the possible side-effects of vaccines. If you've already done any amount of research, you will have heard about the printed inserts that come packaged with every vaccine. These inserts list of all of the ingredients and any side-effects that might have appeared during safety testing. If you haven't read the chapter about vaccine safety, I'd go read that right now. There are a couple of things you need to understand first.

I've avoided talking about side-effects because they can freak people out and prevent them from thinking logically about the cost-benefit of vaccines. I hope by now you'll realize that many of the diseases pediatric vaccines try to protect us from were trivial infections, decades ago, and that was before we really understood how to treat them. Many of the infections that had extremely high death tolls a hundred years ago were because of the poor sanitation, nutrition and medical treatment of that era. In first world countries, there are very few of these infections that are scary anymore. As I've said before, you're putting your child in far more danger just by placing them in their car seat and driving to the doctor's office.

Back to the side-effects—they happen, all the time. They are much more common than most people realize. Many parents don't notice them until days after their kids got their shots and don't even make the connection vaccines may have had something to do with it. My son was two-months old at his first Thanksgiving. We'd traveled to my hometown to be with family, and he wouldn't stop screaming. For hours and hours he screamed and wouldn't eat or sleep. It got so bad I threw up from stress. We didn't know what to do. Maybe he was tired from visiting too many people. Maybe he was getting over a cold, but there wasn't a runny nose or anything else to indicate he was sick. It wasn't until years later we looked back at his shot record and realized he had been given seven shots two days earlier. We have a name for this screaming now—we call it the *encephalitis scream*. His brain was likely swelling so badly it was causing him tremendous pain. If I would have known what to look for, I could have put my thumb on the fontanelle on the top of his head and would have realized it wasn't soft anymore but bulging with pressure from a swollen brain.

Some do make the connection, call the doctor's office, and talk to a nurse who will inevitably tell them something along the lines, "Babies just do that sometimes and we don't know why. Give them some more Tylenol and they should be fine. Wasn't the vaccines, I'm sure of that." If your baby develops significant change after any other medicine, like a rash after antibiotics, your doctor will advise you stop taking them. Vaccines are almost never blamed for these problems. Physicians don't have any other option for disease prevention, so they're more aggressively defended than other medicines. There's always another antibiotic they can try if one seems to cause you problems. If you become afraid of vaccines, they're out of magic tricks.

As you look through the list of vaccine side effects, you will see all sorts of things like *seizures, encephalitis, Guillain-Barre syndrome, thrombocytopenia, Stevens-Johnson syndrome,* vision problems, etc. Thankfully, these more serious complications are rare, but unfortunately, they're not as rare as people think. As I said earlier, one reason is many parents don't make the connection that a vaccine might have caused the problem. If they do and call it in to the doctor's office, they are usually blown off as being paranoid about vaccines. There is a national database that's supposed to catalog these kinds of reactions—It's called VAERS (for Vaccine Adverse Event Reporting System) but most doctors don't even know about it. Because of this, even the real serious reactions that parents *and* their doctors suspect were caused by vaccines don't even get logged in the VAERS database. So there's no reliable record of how often it happens. As you become familiar with what to look for, you'll start to realize how common these side-effects are.

The reality about many of these side effects is any of them can happen if the conditions are right. I don't associate a particular side effect with a particular vaccine—I just know that with any vaccine I'm taking the risk of a number of different problems. I basically categorize vaccine side effects into two groups: neurological and autoimmune. We know your kid's arm or leg is going to hurt like crazy after most shots—I'm not talking about that. I'm talking about neurological side-effects that can affect your brain function and nervous system. They might cause swelling of your brain which will cause your baby to scream with pain. Some people report this when their child received many vaccines at once, like ours did, while I've heard of others that received just one vaccine and developed the same problem. They might cause problems with your brainstem, like cranial nerve dysfunction. This is easily seen with asymmetrical smiles or frowns or misaligned eyes. Read the chapter called "How To Recognize Vaccine Injuries" for more information on that. I'm also talking about some other issues common to vaccine side effects—auto-immune related disorders, something those of us who research vaccines are beginning to believe is a direct result of the aluminum many of them contain.

The problem with all of these side effects is that modern medicine isn't able to treat them very well. There are medicines to reduce the seizures of epilepsy or the inflammation of autoimmune disease, but in terms of cures, there is really nothing—it can be a lifelong battle. For the infections vaccines are supposed to prevent, medicine has gotten really proficient at treating those. Most people can deal with the infection naturally, but if you need help, it's certainly there. I wouldn't get hung up on which vaccines can produce specific side effects—after talking to a lot of parents about their experience, it seems like any vaccine is capable of producing nearly any side effect. Again—thankfully a rare occurrence, but not as rare as those in charge would like you to believe.

Chapter 46
Can Your Children Be Taken From You?

You may have heard of stories of medical kidnapping, where parents have their children taken away from them for refusing to vaccinate. While this does happen, it is very rare, and in most cases is illegal. Although I wouldn't be afraid of this happening, I want to explain why it sometimes does.

If you haven't realized this already, vaccines can be a contentious topic for people. This is especially true for some medical professionals. Vaccines are like their holy grail of treatments, and for parents to question them can hurt their feelings. Some people deal with this fine, while others can get really offended. Sometimes, you, as a new mother, might feel very passionately about skipping the hepatitis B vaccine for your one-hour-old infant. You should—it's a stupid shot that is dangerous and completely unnecessary 99.99% of the time. But the maternity nurse who is tending to you and your newborn may not feel this way. She may not take kindly to you saying the shot is stupid and no one should get it. In fact, she may get angry enough that she threatens you with the biggest weapon in her arsenal—calling in child protective services—because she says you are abusing your child. They have absolutely no legal basis for this, but nothing is stopping them from saying it, because many new mothers don't know better.

You may get angry from that threat and push back by saying something equally stupid like, "I dare you," or "Go ahead, call them right up. They won't do anything." You have just escalated the situation when it should have been *deescalated*. The same thing happens occasionally with police officers. They might have had a really bad day, and/or you might be an especially annoying person to them, and if you say the wrong thing, you can add tension into a situation where they're doing something wrong just because they're mad at you and feel like they have more power than you and can probably get away with it.

Because of this, I would always deescalate the situation. Swallow your pride. Everyone has bad days now and then and lashing out at someone or attacking their authority—possibly the only thing of value they have in their life—may make a minor conflict go south quickly. As I mentioned in an earlier chapter, don't get in arguments or debates in these situations. Explain to them this is a personal decision you've made. If they're super aggressive, ask them for safety studies that show that particular vaccine has been properly tested in infants. Buy yourself some time to cool down. Act curious. Tell them you need more information. Don't try to tell them they are wrong. This will make them angry and more likely to do something stupid, like call CPS on you to try and prove a point.

As far as I know, there is no situation where you can refuse vaccines and have your children taken from you, at least in the United States—legally. It happens, occasionally, but as far as I know, is usually because a health professional acted very unprofessionally and let the vaccine debate get way too personal. Don't do that. Stay cool. Win the debate somewhere else. Let them think they know more than you or alternatively, tell them you discuss medical matters with the doctor only. Move on, and keep things simple.

Chapter 47
How To Recognize Vaccine Injuries

There are a few obvious ways to recognize if something bad has happened to your child after vaccination. Most mothers could count every hair on their baby's head and know right away that something has changed. Eating habits, personality changes, or sleeping patterns—there are a number of things that sometimes feel different after vaccination. You're purposefully injecting your child with a modified version of a disease, so it's natural to expect them to feel bad. Sometimes their arm or leg will be swollen and extremely sensitive to touch. This often happens after injections that contain aluminum as their body forms granulomas or nodules around the metal to keep it from reaching somewhere more dangerous.

You're likely able to recognize any of these signs without any sort of formal training. There are other issues that most mothers wouldn't recognize, even though they're literally staring them in the face. These are the ones I want to mention really quickly because they are indicators your baby may have been neurologically affected by vaccines—something we hope never happens—but unfortunately it sometimes will.

The first, most obvious sign to look for is in your baby's eyes. They should both be pointed straight ahead, looking in the same direction. Sometimes, the aluminum in the vaccines can travel into their brainstem and cause problems with some of the muscles that control their eyes' movement. If this happens, one might turn inward, or sometimes an eye might deviate outward. Doctors call this *strabismus*, and if it were to happen directly after vaccination—like within a few days—you might want to look into metal detox strategies. You probably already have hundreds of pictures of your child, but if you really want to know for sure if something happened, try to get a video of them, looking at you straight on. Take this video directly before your well-child visit, then take another after their well-child visit if you think you see something off. Having this before-after sequence of videos will help document what might have happened to your child.

Another similar problem is with their mouth. Sometimes you'll notice their frown drooping on one side—this is a common problem. If your baby was born with it, you may have already talked to a neurologist about it. If you've never seen it before, but your baby developed it directly after vaccination, I would definitely start looking into some aluminum detox treatments. Another more common injury is a crooked smile. Take a video of your child before their shots and try to catch them smiling straight-on. It should be symmetrical, with both sides of the corners of their mouth pulling up evenly. You can also notice their smile affect their eyes. When they smile, their cheeks should puff up a bit, causing their eyes to narrow—"happy eyes," we call them. When they lose muscle tone on one side, you might notice one eye looking squinty and the other looking round when they smile. The squinty eye is not the problem—your eyes are supposed to do this. The round eye is actually the problem—it can be a clear indicator your child has lost some muscle function on that side of their face. Take another video of your child's face if you notice something appears to be off after their vaccines—it may come in handy as you work through metal detoxing.

These two things are indicators of problems with what we call cranial nerves, but there are many others to be aware of. Babies who cannot hold their head straight anymore so that it tilts to one side—what it called *torticollis*—if they developed this issue directly after vaccination, you might want to look into it. Children whose eyes start flickering side to side can indicate a problem, as can incomplete or involuntary blinks or facial tics. If your baby appears to suddenly be unable to latch after vaccination, this can indicate paralysis with their tongue. In older children, you might notice them start to have speech problems. If your child suddenly has developed a fear of loud noises or even particular noises that don't seem loud to you but make them very upset, this can be indicative of a cranial nerve problem. Finally, another issue might surface as eating problems in the form of having trouble swallowing. If your baby or child suddenly starts spitting up food or is refusing foods they were previously eating just fine, you might want to take note of this and think about looking into metal detoxification.

Because I feel like these unseen warning signs for neurological damage are so important, I've written an entire book about this phenomenon called *Crooked:Man-made Disease Explained*. If you're more interested in any of the symptoms I have mentioned here, there are many others to look out for, and I encourage you to grab a copy of the book and learn how to be on the lookout for the earliest warning signs of this type of neurological injury.

Chapter 48
Don't 3rd World Countries Need Vaccines?

I want to mention something which recently appeared that made me change much about the way I think about vaccines. I used to think that in first world countries, we could afford to be much more lenient with our vaccine schedules. In first world countries, we enjoy the fruits of highly trained physicians, adequately equipped hospitals, and essentially the latest and greatest in medical care. In addition to that, we have proper sanitation that ensures our water supply is generally free of disease. Our options for good nutrition are plentiful and we typically enjoy a life free from the stress of civil war and political instability. Because of all of these things, I felt like it was much easier for citizens of first world countries to approach vaccination with skepticism. Even if something went wrong, which was unlikely, we would have the infrastructure to quickly address any problems.

On the other hand, I thought that in third world countries vaccinations should be treated differently. They *don't* have access to the medical care we do. Their water supplies and food sources are generally much less regulated than ours. They likely live under political strife or threat of civil war—stress-inducing factors which contribute to disease as much as anything else. Because of all of these things, I thought that, while in the first world it was fairly risk-free for anyone to skip certain vaccines, to do this in the third world might be extremely dangerous.

Something recently changed my mind. A study came out a year or two ago from a doctor named Peter Aaby. He's considered the godfather of vaccination in Africa. He has spent most of his professional career pushing for improved immunization programs on the continent. If you say vaccines and Africa in the same sentence, it would be hard not to picture Dr. Peter Aaby—he is the gold standard of immunization promotion in a continent full of third-world countries. A couple of years ago, he did a study where he followed up on the long-term health benefits of children that had received the DPT vaccine (diphtheria, tetanus and pertussis) and those who had not. Those children who had received the DPT vaccine died from those diseases less than those who had not received it—a statistic which would make it appear the shot had worked. Unfortunately another, troubling, part of the study revealed that those children who received the DPT shot had a *10 times higher* mortality rate overall than those who hadn't received it. The shot seemed to offer them some protection from the three diseases the vaccine was designed for, but on the whole, it was clear, the children's long-term health had suffered. And this wasn't just a tiny difference, this was a jaw-dropping difference in mortality—if you had received the DPT vaccine, you were *10 times* as likely to die than if you had never received it at all. The results of the study were stark enough to give everyone like me a shock. The godfather of vaccines in Africa not only admitted—but *published* a paper—for all to see that showed those who received that particular vaccine had a mortality rate 10 times worse than those who didn't get the shot. For someone whose career was based on African immunization, that was an incredibly humbling discovery, I'm sure.

As I mention elsewhere, the polio vaccine creates its own set of problems, usually in the form of more polio. And knowing that the DPT vaccine in Africa appeared to be so detrimental to those people—it made me begin to rethink everything. I thought skipping or delaying vaccines in first world countries was an option those in third world countries could not afford to make. After that paper came out, I began to have my doubts.

Chapter 49
Should You Be Worried About Zika?

You probably remember hearing a lot about the Zika story that happened in Brazil a couple of years ago and the mysterious birth defects that seemed to be caused by it. I think I know exactly what caused the huge spike in children with birth defects and I want to share it with you because I don't think you have anything to worry about from Zika. The reason these children's lives were ruined was entirely preventable, and I think we should ask what caused it so that we might avoid doing it again.

Just to refresh your memory, in 2015, there was a huge spike in reported cases of women having children with birth defects—most commonly, microcephaly, which is when babies are born with a very small head. There were thousands of these babies—it was a *huge* spike that alarmed everyone. When they discovered that many of these pregnant women had contracted the recently imported Zika virus during their pregnancy, they were understandably *very* concerned.

It appeared that the Zika virus was causing children to develop birth defects. Governments all over the world went into a panic and were begging for money to develop a vaccine. Cities like Miami were being carpet-bombed with pesticides known to cause birth defects, and people were getting abortions, skipping the Olympics in Brazil—all kinds of things because of the dire warnings about Zika. But then an interesting thing happened—the birth defects seemed to stop. They didn't disappear completely, but nearly did. They went from thousands that summer and fall of 2015 almost back to zero in 2016—back to where they were before, at the very least. No one could figure out what happened. The media, had been playing messages of alarm. They were being told by authorities that Zika was causing birth defects and it appeared to be spreading. But something changed. The media went silent. No more Zika stories. No more Zika questions.

What happened? What caused all the birth defects in Brazil in 2015? First off, part of it's based on the fact that we've recently discovered that aluminum travels around the body inside white blood cells. Remember that white blood cells are the frontline defense of your immune system. So if you have aluminum in your body *and* you have an area with inflammation, that area is going to get this neurotoxin. Got it?

The Zika virus is attracted to neural stem cells. Neural stem cells are important to the development of not just the fetal brain, but the entire central nervous system, possibly even more. There are lots of neural stem cells in a developing fetus. Secondly, the virus had apparently mutated in some form to cause a more infectious strain sometime before a small 2013 outbreak in French Polynesia. A more infectious strain *might* provide a cause for the increase in Zika infections, and the neural stem cell phenomenon *might* explain how Zika could cause neurological development problems, but it *didn't* explain the sudden spike of birth defects in 2015—this was a *massive* increase. And it didn't explain its sudden disappearance in 2016. People were still getting Zika infections in other countries, but the birth defects weren't happening there—it was just Brazil.

In 2014, a technical report was issued nationwide by the Brazilian Health Department's Immunization Division. In October of that year, Brazilian health officials issued a new rule: Pertussis, also known as whooping cough, was shaping up to be a big problem and they were recommending the shot be given for all pregnant women. But there was an ominous part of the bulletin that should have concerned any physician reading it. For any woman not vaccinated previously for pertussis, the bulletin recommended: "Administer the first two doses of the shot and the last dose of shot between the 27th and preferably up to the 36th week of gestation." They were recommending pregnant women receive up to *three* doses of this shot—each one containing up to .4 mg of aluminum.

The doctors, it would appear, took the memo seriously. PBS Frontline did an interview with several mothers in Brazil whose babies had developed microcephaly. They said "an 18-year-old mother of a child recently diagnosed with microcephaly, is inclined to believe vaccines may be the problem. She says she never had symptoms of Zika, but she did receive a shot from her public health clinic *every month* of her pregnancy. As she waited for an appointment at the public hospital in Recife, she tried to soothe her fussing baby, but said she couldn't recall exactly what the shots were for." I can only hope she didn't actually receive a vaccine every month of her pregnancy, but from the unease of other mothers around her at this time and area, you can tell there were a lot of shots given.

The mother also didn't recall having anything resembling a Zika infection at all—unsurprising given the innocuous nature of the virus. Knowing that most of these 2015 microcephaly cases appeared in a specific region of Brazil, amongst some of the poorest mothers in that area, one could see how their vaccination status might fall into the "unknown" category. It's also not hard to imagine a recently inspired doctor wanting to be extra-sure the mother's baby wouldn't have to suffer a pertussis infection and erring on the "safe" side by administering the three-shot course of injections—just in case. Hopefully the 18-year old mother's memory was faulty and they stopped at just three shots.

What do I think happened? I believe that Zika virus infections actually *did* surface in a very particular area—northeastern Brazil in 2014—the same area where the birth defects started happening. This is what threw them off. It was relatively unknown to South America until this time. In other areas of the world with previous infections, Zika had been an innocuous virus that wasn't associated with microcephaly. It was a new disease, and was fanning out just like you might expect any other infection to spread. But a Zika infection alone is not what actually created the microcephaly. It needed something else—a neurotoxin—to do it.

Zika turns out to be a peculiar infection because it appears to cause in inflammation in the fetal brain, something the maternal and fetal immune system apparently can cope with under normal circumstances—as evidenced by a *lack* of birth defects associated with Zika more often than not. You may have heard that vaccines have not been adequately safety tested on pregnant women. Even if they were, we can be sure the safety tests would not have permitted administering 3 or more doses during one pregnancy. The 2014 Brazilian memo came at the worst possible time for some. It was a national roll-out and there were undoubtedly mothers across the country that received multiple doses of the TDaP vaccine during their pregnancy. For a very unlucky group of women—those who received multiple injections of aluminum *and* got a Zika infection at the same time, their children were likely to suffer greatly.

From what we know about the infection, it's likely to have created inflammation in the neural stem cells of the fetal brain. Again, with a properly functioning immune system, most babies could evidently make it through unscathed. However, with their white blood cells full of aluminum, it's unsurprising when these poor children's immune systems asked for help, they received a neurotoxic response.

The technical memo about vaccinating pregnant women with three DTaP vaccines is now gone from the Brazilian Health Department's site—it has completely disappeared, and I had to use special tools to find an archived version. There is no reference to this program or any recommendations that I can find regarding pregnant women and this vaccine. And in a final note of irony, I realized the memo was released in October 2014. Exactly ten months later, in August of 2015, the first cases of birth defects began to appear in Brazil. It would seem that Zika, without the aluminum injections, is a minor illness. Apparently, the Brazilian health officials who removed all references to this health memo would agree, even if they don't fully understand what happened.

So to answer your question, no, you don't need to worry about Zika. I'd be much more worried about the pesticides they're trying to spray in your neighborhood to control mosquitoes than the infection itself.

Chapter 50
Closing

It can feel frightening to contemplate skipping vaccines for your children. We've been told our whole lives that they are the only thing standing in between certain death and a lifetime of happiness. Unfortunately, the reality is much, much different. Vaccines can be a barbaric practice and I believe they might be considered a medical relic within a few decades. Imagine restraining your children on a table and purposefully injecting them with modified disease. Take away the linoleum floor, the fluorescent lights and blue scrubs. In any other setting, this practice might feel like a Satanic ritual. For some reason, we have grown to accept this as a natural and acceptable process to put our children through.

In the United States, children are made to undergo this procedure dozens of times—often times kicking and screaming the whole way, requiring multiple nurses to pin them down. All in hopes the vaccine might protect them from a disease they might get that most of humanity never feared before the vaccines. It's truly insane—from my perspective, at least.

Knowing that most diseases ceased to be dangerous long before vaccines arrived on the scene, knowing that the appearance and disappearance of polio coincided perfectly with some extremely dangerous pesticides that were often sprayed directly onto children, and knowing that vaccines are so poorly safety tested and contain ingredients I'd never let my children ingest (let alone be injected into them), not vaccinating is a very easy decision.

I am not ignorant to the danger of certain infections. I have studied them and respect the harm they can sometimes cause. I also have faith that modern medicine could take care of things if something bad happened. Finally, I am very suspicious that the ingredients in vaccines are responsible for many of the new neurological and auto-immune conditions that have appeared over the last 100 years.

Think about this—let's say a company had a new product to sell you. It was a special cage you could place around your child's crib that would most likely prevent them from being struck by lightning. But there's a catch—the material the cage is made from can be toxic to some children and cause them some nasty side effects. The side effects are rare, though. Most children seem to be fine, and you can sleep comfortably knowing they would be protected from lightning strikes while they slept. Would you buy it? Are you so concerned about lightning strikes you would buy this contraption and risk them having a reaction to it? Most people wouldn't, and it's understandable why. The reality is, the chance of a being struck by lightning—at one in 700,000—is much more likely than an infection from most of these illnesses. They are extremely rare, and even with an infection, it's uncommon that something bad would happen. You probably put your child to bed every night and never think a thought about them being struck by lightning. But because we have vaccines available to us, they make us worry, instead of feeling comforted. Strange how they work like that, isn't it?

As a result, I personally would *currently* forego all vaccines listed on the United States CDC schedule for my children. Every one of them. You may go on to skip the polio vaccine, or one or two of the others, or you may go on to follow the Dutch or Swedish vaccine schedule, but whatever your choice, the research you do now will no doubt improve the future health of your children. Unfortunately, you cannot trust the information that comes from most health care providers or government health officials. They don't mean any harm to your children, but if history is any guide, they will be the very last to admit vaccines are causing serious problems.

This very minute, these two groups are recommending pregnant women get the flu and TDaP shots, even though they haven't been safety tested in pregnant women. The TDaP shot they recommend contains a large amount of aluminum, something you would never willingly allow into your developing fetus for any other reason. This one recommendation, which your doctor will also strongly suggest despite there having been no safety tests performed, should be a strong indicator of the recklessness with which health care providers treat vaccines.

The hepatitis B vaccine they will try to inject in your newborn —for a disease they're unlikely to get (unless you test positive for it) —contains a large amount of aluminum. Other countries *don't* recommend this vaccine. I would consider looking into skipping this vaccine. It is a needless risk for such a young infant.

Finally, I feel that I have to warn you about a few things. You may have already sensed this, but if you do begin to question vaccines, you should be ready to be treated very differently. Many physicians know little about vaccines, yet hold them in a revered place above all other medicines. If you question any of their knowledge on vaccines, or give any indication you may be suspicious about their safety, be prepared to be treated poorly.

I wish that I could say doctors and nurses always respond positively to these questions and concerns, but they sometimes react very poorly. Most pediatricians receive generous kickbacks from insurance companies—so long as all of their patients are fully vaccinated. If the percent of their fully vaccinated patients drops below a certain number, they can lose their entire compensation. As a result, doctors (and their nurses) are very aggressive about vaccinating every child that walks through the door, even if they are clearly sick and should be nowhere near a vaccine.

Many pediatric practices will "fire" you if you do not follow their vaccination program perfectly. They will claim they are doing this out of a concern for the safety of the other patients at the clinic. This is not true. Most are simply trying to protect the generous kickbacks they get from insurance companies. If you are going to cause problems by skipping or delaying certain vaccines, you might cost them hundreds of thousands of dollars.

Because of this, many parents go to a family doctor or pediatric chiropractor for check-ups. These physicians don't normally have the kickback programs hanging over their heads and aren't as aggressive about forcing needless vaccines on your family. If you don't already know this, the pediatric "well visits" that doctors request your baby for are really just shot visits. Nurses will weigh them, measure, and check some other development milestones, but it's nothing you couldn't do yourself at home.

New parents are nervous and feel like they have to see a doctor every few weeks just to make sure everything is okay, but the reality is these visits are to facilitate more vaccines and little else. They will really push these visits hard. If you interview a pediatric doctor, tell them you're not interested in the first year of well visit checkups—just to see their reaction. Tell them you'll come to them if your child is sick (a novel concept, I realize) and nothing else. You may be surprised at their reaction.

If it is legal to do so, I would use the audio recorder function on your phone and record your interactions with your doctor or nurse. It may be helpful after you meet with them to review what they told you, especially if anything they said was in a threatening tone.

This is an unfortunate reality of having children within the context of a modern medical system. If you don't play along completely with the vaccine game, you will be a square peg in a round hole and will have to learn the best ways to present yourself. I hate things are this way. I remember when most doctors and nurses were happy to listen to your concerns and respect your maternal instincts about what medical procedures were appropriate for your children. Thankfully, more and more of them are beginning to research vaccines just like you or I are doing. That means this won't be difficult forever.

As I mentioned earlier, I've just scratched the surface on the truth about vaccines. There are many other things I haven't addressed which you can find out about as you do more research on the subject. Whatever you do, I wish the best for you and your family and truly hope you are able to have happy, healthy lives free of neurological, chronic and autoimmune disease. It is my prayer, as I said in the first chapter, that we "Let no innocent life in our city be quenched again in useless pain through our ignorance and sin." Thank you for reading, and I hope this book helped you in some way.

About the Author

FORREST MAREADY IS A HISTORIAN, RESEARCHER AND author who has spent the last few years of his life focusing on the underlying causes of the neurological, autoimmune, and chronic illnesses of the modern age. His book, *The Autism Vaccine*, tells the incredible story of how a new childhood vaccine developed in the 1930s first became associated with autism.

His book, *Crooked:Man-made Disease Explained* chronicles the medicinal metals—mercury and arsenic—of the 1800s, and how they became even more insidious as aluminum and mercury began to be injected directly into the body at the turn of the century.

The Moth in the Iron Lung tells how an invasive species escaped from Boston, Massachusetts, and a new pesticide invented to stop its spread led to the deadly outbreaks of polio across the Northeastern, United States at that time.

Maready spent much of his professional career working in the film and television industries as an editor, sound engineer, animator, and composer. He attended Wake Forest University and lives along the beaches of coastal North Carolina.

Other popular books by Forrest Maready:

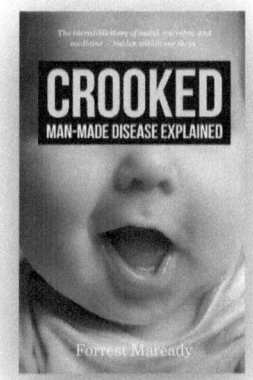

Crooked:
The incredible story of metal, microbes, and medicine—hidden with our faces.

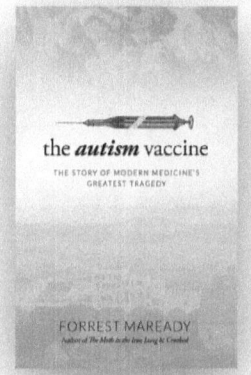

The Autism Vaccine:
The story of modern medicine's greatest tragedy.

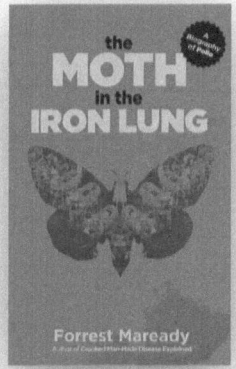

The Moth in the Iron Lung:
The story of polio that explains everything.

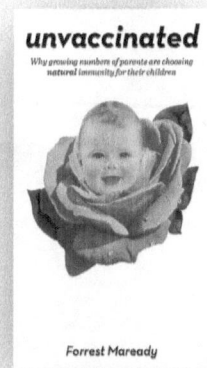

Unvaccinated:
Why parents are choosing natural immunity.

Available at select retailers and:
www.**forrestmaready**.com

www.ingramcontent.com/pod-product-compliance
Lightning Source LLC
Chambersburg PA
CBHW032000170526
45157CB00002B/480